GRAPHING CALCULATOR MANUAL

JUDITH A. PENNA

Indiana University Purdue University Indianapolis

WITH THE ASSISTANCE OF
DAPHNE A. BELL

INTERMEDIATE ALGEBRA
GRAPHS & MODELS

SECOND EDITION

Marvin L. Bittinger

Indiana University Purdue University Indianapolis

David J. Ellenbogen

Community College of Vermont

Barbara L. Johnson

Indiana University Purdue University Indianapolis

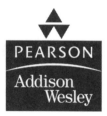

PEARSON

Addison
Wesley

Boston   San Francisco   New York
London   Toronto   Sydney   Tokyo   Singapore   Madrid
Mexico City   Munich   Paris   Cape Town   Hong Kong   Montreal

Copyright © 2004 Pearson Education, Inc.
Publishing as Pearson Addison-Wesley, 75 Arlington Street, Boston MA 02116

ISBN   0-321-16863-1

2 3 4 5 6 VHG 06 05 04 03

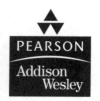

Contents

The TI-83 and TI-83 Plus
Graphics Calculators

Chapter 1
Basics of Algebra and Graphing

GETTING STARTED

Press $\boxed{\text{ON}}$ to turn on the TI-83 or TI-83 Plus graphing calculator. ($\boxed{\text{ON}}$ is the key at the bottom left-hand corner of the keypad.) You should see a blinking rectangle, or cursor, on the screen. If you do not see the cursor, try adjusting the display contrast. To do this, first press $\boxed{\text{2nd}}$. ($\boxed{\text{2nd}}$ is the yellow key in the left column of the keypad.) Then press and hold $\boxed{\triangle}$ to increase the contrast or $\boxed{\triangledown}$ to decrease the contrast.

To turn the calculator off, press $\boxed{\text{2nd}}$ $\boxed{\text{OFF}}$. (OFF is the second operation associated with the $\boxed{\text{ON}}$ key.) The calculator will turn itself off automatically after about five minutes without any activity.

Press $\boxed{\text{MODE}}$ to display the MODE settings. Initially you should select the settings on the left side of the display.

To change a setting on the Mode screen use $\boxed{\triangledown}$ or $\boxed{\triangle}$ to move the cursor to the line of that setting. Then use $\boxed{\triangleright}$ or $\boxed{\triangleleft}$ to move the blinking cursor to the desired setting and press $\boxed{\text{ENTER}}$. Press $\boxed{\text{CLEAR}}$ or $\boxed{\text{2nd}}$ $\boxed{\text{QUIT}}$ to leave the MODE screen. (QUIT is the second operation associated with the $\boxed{\text{MODE}}$ key.) Pressing $\boxed{\text{CLEAR}}$ or $\boxed{\text{2nd}}$ $\boxed{\text{QUIT}}$ will take you to the home screen where computations are performed.

The TI-83 and TI-83 Plus graphing calculators are very similar in many respects. For that reason, most of the keystrokes and instructions presented in this section of the graphing calculator manual will apply to both calculators. Where they differ, keystrokes and instructions for using the TI-83 will be given first, followed by those for the TI-83 Plus.

It will be helpful to read the Introduction to the Graphing Calculator on pages 9 and 10 of your textbook as well as the Getting Started section of your graphing calculator Guidebook before proceeding.

ORDER OF OPERATIONS

The TI-83 and TI-83 Plus follow the rules for order of operations.

Section 1.1, Example 9 Evaluate $2(y-3)^2 + 7$ for $y = 5$.

Enter the expression on the home screen, substituting 5 for y. Press 2 $\boxed{(}$ 5 $\boxed{-}$ 3 $\boxed{)}$ $\boxed{x^2}$ $\boxed{+}$ 7 $\boxed{\text{ENTER}}$. Note that the blue

$-$ key in the right-hand column of the keypad is the subtraction key. The $(-)$ key on the bottom row of the keypad represents "the opposite of" or "the additive inverse of" rather than subtraction. In the expression above we could also have squared $(5-3)$ by pressing $\wedge$ 2 rather than x^2. The $\wedge$ key indicates exponentiation and the number following it indicates the exponent.

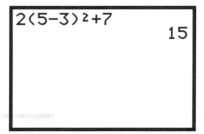

You can recall and edit your entry if necessary. If, for instance, in the expression above you pressed 8 instead of 5, first press 2nd ENTRY to return to the last entry. (ENTRY is the second operation associated with the ENTER key.) Then use the $\triangleleft$ key to move the cursor to 8 and press 5 to overwrite it. If you forgot to type the left parenthesis, move the cursor to the 5; then press 2nd INS (to insert the parenthesis before the 5. (INS is the second operation associated with the DEL key.) You can continue to insert symbols immediately after the first insertion without pressing 2nd INS again. If you typed 21 instead of 2, move the cursor to 1 and press DEL. This will delete the 1. If you notice that an entry needs to be edited before you press ENTER to perform the computation, the editing can be done directly without recalling the entry.

The keystrokes 2nd ENTRY can be used repeatedly to recall entries preceding the last one. Pressing 2nd ENTRY twice, for example, will recall the next to last entry. Using these keystrokes a third time recalls the third to last entry and so on. The number of entries that can be recalled depends on the amount of storage they occupy in the calculator's memory.

USING A MENU

A menu is a list of options that appears when a key is pressed. Thus, multiple options, and sometimes multiple menus, may be accessed by pressing one key. For example, the following screen appears when the MATH key is pressed. We see four submenus, MATH, NUM, CPX, and PRB as well as the options in the MATH submenu.

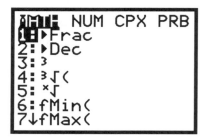

We can copy an item from a menu to the home screen either by using the up or down arrow key to highlight its number and then pressing ENTER or by simply pressing the number of the item. The down-arrow beside item 7 in the menu above indicates that there are additional items in the menu. Use the $\triangledown$ key to scroll down to them.

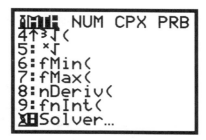

The next example involves both order of operations and choosing an option from a menu.

Section 1.2, Example 13 Calculate: $\dfrac{14 - 3| - 16 + 38|}{4| - 2^4 - 3^2|}$.

In order to divide the entire numerator of this fraction by the entire denominator, we must enclose both the numerator and the denominator in parentheses. Recall also that the $\boxed{(-)}$ key in the bottom row of the keypad must be used to enter a negative number on the calculator whereas the blue $\boxed{-}$ key is used to enter subtraction. On the TI-83 and TI-83 Plus, $|x|$ is written abs(X). Absolute value notation is item 1 on the MATH NUM menu.

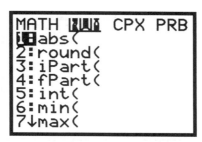

To enter the expression above, press $\boxed{(}$ 1 4 $\boxed{-}$ 3 $\boxed{\text{MATH}}$ $\boxed{\triangleright}$ $\boxed{\text{ENTER}}$ $\boxed{(-)}$ 1 6 $\boxed{+}$ 3 8 $\boxed{)}$ $\boxed{)}$ $\boxed{\div}$ $\boxed{(}$ 4 $\boxed{\text{MATH}}$ $\boxed{\triangleright}$ $\boxed{\text{ENTER}}$ $\boxed{(-)}$ 2 $\boxed{\wedge}$ 4 $\boxed{-}$ 3 $\boxed{x^2}$ $\boxed{)}$ $\boxed{)}$ $\boxed{\text{ENTER}}$.

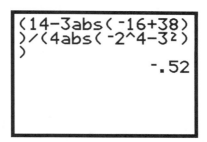

Note that the calculator supplies the left parenthesis in the absolute value notation. The absolute value expression must be closed with a right parenthesis which must be entered manually. The second right parenthesis in the numerator serves, along with the first left parenthesis, to enclose the entire numerator in parentheses. This is done in the denominator as well.

Instead of pressing $\boxed{\text{MATH}}$ $\boxed{\triangleright}$ $\boxed{\text{ENTER}}$ to access "abs(" and copy it to the home screen, we could have pressed $\boxed{\text{MATH}}$ $\boxed{\triangleright}$ 1 since "abs(" is item 1 on the MATH NUM menu. Absolute value notation can also be found as the first item in the CATALOG and copied to the home screen. To do this press $\boxed{\text{2nd}}$ $\boxed{\text{CATALOG}}$ $\boxed{\text{ENTER}}$. (CATALOG is the second operation associated with the 0 numeric key.)

The result of the calculation above can be converted from decimal notation to fractional notation by pressing $\boxed{\text{MATH}}$ $\boxed{\text{ENTER}}$ $\boxed{\text{ENTER}}$ or $\boxed{\text{MATH}}$ 1 $\boxed{\text{ENTER}}$. These keystrokes tell the calculator to use the previous answer, and then they access the MATH MATH menu, copy item 1 "▷ Frac" to the home screen, and display the conversion. Note that this must be done immediately after the calculation is performed in order to have the result of the calculation available for the conversion.

```
(14-3abs( -16+38)
)/(4abs( -2^4-3²)
)
               -.52
Ans▶Frac
             -13/25
■
```

If only a fractional answer is desired, the keystrokes $\boxed{\text{MATH}}$ $\boxed{\text{ENTER}}$ or $\boxed{\text{MATH}}$ 1 can be inserted before the final $\boxed{\text{ENTER}}$ in the computation and a fractional answer will be displayed immediately.

```
(14-3abs( -16+38)
)/(4abs( -2^4-3²)
)▶Frac
             -13/25
■
```

SCIENTIFIC NOTATION

To enter a number in scientific notation, first type the decimal portion of the number; then press $\boxed{\text{2nd}}$ $\boxed{\text{EE}}$ (EE is the second operation associated with the $\boxed{,}$ key.); finally type the exponent, which can be at most two digits. For example, to enter 1.789×10^{-11} in scientific notation, press 1 $\boxed{.}$ 7 8 9 $\boxed{\text{2nd}}$ $\boxed{\text{EE}}$ $\boxed{(-)}$ 1 1 $\boxed{\text{ENTER}}$. To enter 6.084×10^{23} in scientific notation, press 6 $\boxed{.}$ 0 8 4 $\boxed{\text{2nd}}$ $\boxed{\text{EE}}$ 2 3 $\boxed{\text{ENTER}}$. The decimal portion of each number appears before a small E while the exponent follows the E.

```
1.789E-11
           1.789E-11
6.084E23
          6.084E23
```

The graphing calculator can be used to perform computations in scientific notation.

Section 1.4, Example 14 Use a graphing calculator to check the computation $(7.2 \times 10^5)(4.3 \times 10^9) = 3.096 \times 10^{15}$.

We enter the computation in scientific notation. Press 7 $\boxed{.}$ 2 $\boxed{\text{2nd}}$ $\boxed{\text{EE}}$ 5 $\boxed{\times}$ 4 $\boxed{.}$ 3 $\boxed{\text{2nd}}$ $\boxed{\text{EE}}$ 9 $\boxed{\text{ENTER}}$. We have 3.096×10^{15}, which checks.

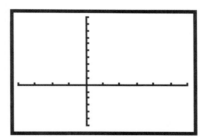

SETTING THE VIEWING WINDOW

The viewing window is the portion of the coordinate plane that appears on the calculator's screen. It is defined by the minimum and maximum values of x and y: Xmin, Xmax, Ymin, and Ymax. The notation [Xmin, Xmax, Ymin, Ymax] is used in the text to represent these window settings or dimensions. For example, $[-12, 12, -8, 8]$ denotes a window that displays the portion of the x-axis from -12 to 12 and the portion of the y-axis from -8 to 8. In addition, the distance between tick marks on the axes is defined by the settings Xscl and Yscl. In this manual Xscl and Yscl will be assumed to be 1 unless noted otherwise. The setting Xres sets the pixel resolution. We usually select Xres = 1. The window corresponding to the settings $[-20, 30, -12, 20]$, Xscl = 5, Yscl = 2, Xres = 1, is shown below.

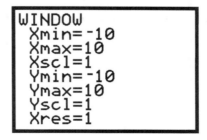

Press the $\boxed{\text{WINDOW}}$ key on the top row of the keypad to display the current window settings on your graphing calculator. The standard settings are shown below.

```
WINDOW
 Xmin=-10
 Xmax=10
 Xscl=1
 Ymin=-10
 Ymax=10
 Yscl=1
 Xres=1
```

To change a setting, position the cursor beside the setting you wish to change and enter the new value. For example, to change from the standard settings to $[-20, \ 30, \ -12, \ 20]$, Xscl = 5, Yscl = 2, on the WINDOW screen press $\boxed{(-)}$ 2 0 $\boxed{\text{ENTER}}$ 3 0 $\boxed{\text{ENTER}}$ 5 $\boxed{\text{ENTER}}$ $\boxed{(-)}$ 1 2 $\boxed{\text{ENTER}}$ 2 0 $\boxed{\text{ENTER}}$ 2 $\boxed{\text{ENTER}}$. The $\boxed{\triangledown}$ key may be used instead of $\boxed{\text{ENTER}}$ after typing each window setting. To see the window shown on the previous page, press the $\boxed{\text{GRAPH}}$ key on the top row of the keypad.

QUICK TIP: To return quickly to the standard window setting $[-10, \ 10, \ -10, \ 10]$, Xscl = 1, Yscl = 1, press $\boxed{\text{ZOOM}}$ 6.

GRAPHING EQUATIONS

After entering an equation and setting a viewing window, you can view the graph of an equation.

Section 1.5, Example 5 Graph $y = 2x$ using a graphing calculator.

Equations are entered on the equation-editor screen. Press $\boxed{\text{Y} =}$ to access this screen. If any of Plot 1, Plot 2, and Plot 3 is turned on (highlighted), turn it off by using the arrow keys to move the blinking cursor over the plot name and pressing $\boxed{\text{ENTER}}$. If there is currently an expression displayed for Y_1, clear it by positioning the cursor beside "$Y_1 =$" and press $\boxed{\text{CLEAR}}$. Do the same for expressions that appear on all other lines by using $\boxed{\triangledown}$ to move to a line and then pressing $\boxed{\text{CLEAR}}$. Then use $\boxed{\triangle}$ or $\boxed{\triangledown}$ to move the cursor to the top line beside "$Y_1 =$." Now press 2 $\boxed{\text{X, T, } \Theta, n}$ to enter the right-hand side of the equation in the Y = screen.

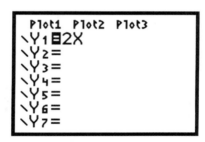

The standard $[-10, 10, -10, 10]$ window is a good choice for this graph. Either enter these dimensions in the WINDOW screen and then press $\boxed{\text{GRAPH}}$ to see the graph or simply press $\boxed{\text{ZOOM}}$ 6 to select the standard window and see the graph.

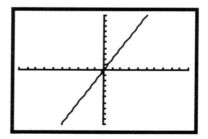

THE TABLE FEATURE

For an equation entered in the equation-editor screen, a table of x-and y-values can be displayed.

Section 1.5, Example 7 Create a table of ordered pairs that are solutions of the equation $y = -\frac{1}{2}x$. Use integer values of x beginning at -3.

First press $\boxed{Y =}$ to access the equation-editor screen. Then clear any equations that are present. (See Example 5 above for the procedure to follow.) Next enter the equation by positioning the cursor beside "$Y_1 =$" and pressing $\boxed{(-)}$ $\boxed{(}$ $\boxed{1}$ $\boxed{\div}$ $\boxed{2}$ $\boxed{)}$ $\boxed{X, T, \Theta, n}$. Although the parentheses are not necessary on the TI-83 and TI-83 Plus, the equation is more easily read when they are used.

Once the equation in entered, press $\boxed{\text{2nd}}$ $\boxed{\text{TBLSET}}$ to display the table set-up screen. (TBLSET is the second function associated with the $\boxed{\text{WINDOW}}$ key.) You can choose to supply the x-values yourself or you can set the calculator to supply them. If "Indpnt" is set to "Auto," the calculator will supply values for x, beginning with the value specified as TblStart and continuing by adding the value of ΔTbl to the preceding value for x. For the equation $y = -\frac{1}{2}x$ entered above, we will set the table to Auto mode and display a table of values that starts with $x = -3$ and adds 1 to the preceding x-value. Press -3 $\boxed{\triangledown}$ 1 to select a minimum x-value of -3 and an increment of 1. The "Indpnt" and "Depend" settings should both be "Auto." If either is not, use the $\boxed{\triangledown}$ key to position the blinking cursor over "Auto" on that line and then press $\boxed{\text{ENTER}}$. To display the table press $\boxed{\text{2nd}}$ $\boxed{\text{TABLE}}$. (TABLE is the second function associated with the $\boxed{\text{GRAPH}}$ key.)

GRAPHS AS MODELS

A graphing calculator can plot data points and draw a line graph using those points.

Section 1.6, Example 7 *Weekly Newspapers.* The following table show the number of weekly newspapers in the United States for various years from 1960 to 2000. Use the data to draw a line graph.

Year	Number of Weekday Newspapers
1960	8174
1970	7612
1980	7954
1990	7606
2000	7689

We will enter the coordinates of the ordered pairs on the STAT list editor screen. To clear any existing lists press $\boxed{\text{STAT}}$ 4

$\boxed{\text{2nd}}$ $\boxed{\text{L}_1}$ $\boxed{\text{,}}$ $\boxed{\text{2nd}}$ $\boxed{\text{L}_2}$ $\boxed{\text{,}}$ $\boxed{\text{2nd}}$ $\boxed{\text{L}_3}$ $\boxed{\text{,}}$ $\boxed{\text{2nd}}$ $\boxed{\text{L}_4}$ $\boxed{\text{,}}$ $\boxed{\text{2nd}}$ $\boxed{\text{L}_5}$ $\boxed{\text{,}}$ $\boxed{\text{2nd}}$ $\boxed{\text{L}_6}$ $\boxed{\text{ENTER}}$. (L_1 through L_6 are the second operations associated with the numeric keys 1 through 6.) The lists can also be cleared by first accessing the STAT list editor screen by pressing $\boxed{\text{STAT}}$ $\boxed{\text{ENTER}}$ or $\boxed{\text{STAT}}$ 1. These keystrokes display the STAT EDIT menu and then select the Edit option from that menu. Then, for each list that contains entries, use the arrow keys to move the cursor to highlight the name of the list at the top of the column and press $\boxed{\text{CLEAR}}$ $\boxed{\triangledown}$ or $\boxed{\text{CLEAR}}$ $\boxed{\text{ENTER}}$.

Once the lists are cleared, we can enter the coordinates of the points. We will enter the first coordinates (x-coordinates) in L_1 and the second coordinates (y-coordinates) in L_2. Position the cursor at the top of column L_1, below the L_1 heading. To enter 1960 press 1 9 6 0 $\boxed{\text{ENTER}}$. Continue entering the x-values 1970, 1980, 1990, and 2000, each followed by $\boxed{\text{ENTER}}$. The entries can be followed by $\boxed{\triangledown}$ rather than $\boxed{\text{ENTER}}$ if desired. Press $\boxed{\triangleright}$ to move to the top of column L_2. Enter the y-values 8174, 7612, 7954, 7606, and 7689 in succession, each followed by $\boxed{\text{ENTER}}$ or $\boxed{\triangledown}$. Note that the coordinates of each point must be in the same position in both lists.

```
L1        L2        L3        2
1960      8174      ------
1970      7612
1980      7954
1990      7606
2000      7689
------
L2(6) =
```

To plot the points, we turn on the STAT PLOT feature. To access the STAT PLOT screen, press $\boxed{\text{2nd}}$ $\boxed{\text{STAT PLOT}}$. (STAT PLOT is the second operation associated with the $\boxed{\text{Y =}}$ key in the upper left-hand corner of the keypad.)

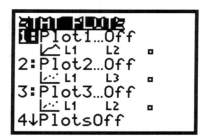

We will use Plot 1. Access it by highlighting 1 and pressing $\boxed{\text{ENTER}}$ or simply by pressing 1. Now position the cursor over On and press $\boxed{\text{ENTER}}$ to turn on Plot 1. The entries Type, Xlist, and Ylist should be as shown below. The last item, Mark, allows us to choose a box, a cross, or a dot for each point. Here we have selected a box. To select Type and Mark, position the cursor over the appropriate selection and press $\boxed{\text{ENTER}}$. Use the L_1 and L_2 keys (associated with the 1 and 2 numeric keys) to select Xlist and Ylist.

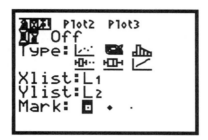

The plot can also be turned on from the "Y =" screen. Press $\boxed{Y =}$, the key at the top left-hand corner of the keypad, to go to this screen. Then, assuming Plot 1 has not yet been turned on, position the cursor over Plot 1 and press $\boxed{\text{ENTER}}$. Plot 1 will now be highlighted.

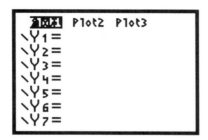

Note that there should be no equations entered on the "Y =" screen. If there are entries present clear them now. (See page 8 of this manual for instructions on clearing equations.) If this is not done, the equations that are currently entered will be graphed along with the data points that are entered.

Now select a viewing window that will display all the data points. The years range from 1960 to 2000 and the numbers newspapers range from 7606 to 8174, so one good choice is [1950, 2010, 7500, 8500], Xscl = 10, Yscl = 100. Press $\boxed{\text{GRAPH}}$ to see the line graph of the data.

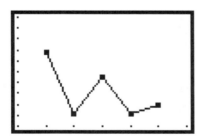

QUICK TIP: Instead of entering the window dimensions directly, we can press $\boxed{\text{ZOOM}}$ 9 after entering the coordinates of the points in lists, turning on Plot 1, and selecting Type, Xlist, Ylist, and Mark. This activates the ZoomStat operation which automatically defines a viewing window that displays all the points and also displays the graph.

Turn off the STAT PLOT as described on page 8 of this manual before graphing other equations.

THE TRACE FEATURE

The graphing calculator's Trace feature displays the coordinates of points of a graph.

Section 1.6, Example 8 *Model Rockets.* Suppose that a model rocket is launched upward with an initial velocity of 96 ft/sec. Its height in feet, h, after t seconds is given by

$$h = -16t^2 + 96t.$$

(a) For how long will the rocket climb?

(b) How high will the rocket go?

(c) After how long will the rocket reach the ground?

First we press $\boxed{Y =}$ to go to the equation-editor screen. Enter $Y_1 = -16x^2 + 96x$ and graph the equation in the viewing window $[0, 10, 0, 200]$, $\text{Yscl} = 10$. Note that the Stat Plots should be turned off. (See page 8 of this manual for the procedure.)

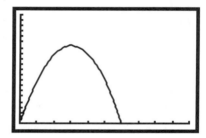

(a) The rocket climbs until the graph reaches the greatest y-value. The x-value associated with this y-value indicates how long the rocket climbs. To find this value, press the $\boxed{\text{TRACE}}$ key in the top row of the keypad. The trace cursor appears on the graph. Use the right and left arrow keys to move the cursor to the highest point on the graph. The greatest y-value occurs when x is about 3, so we can say that the rocket climbs for about 3 seconds.

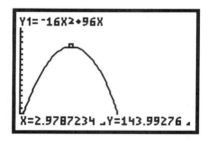

(b) To approximate how high the rocket will go, we read the greatest y-value in the Trace window above. Thus, we would say that the rocket will go to a height of about 144 feet.

(c) The rocket is on the ground when $y = 0$. The x-value associated with this y-value indicates how long it will take the rocket to reach the ground. We use Trace to find this x-value. Press $\boxed{\text{TRACE}}$ and use the right arrow key to move the cursor to the point on the right side of the graph where y is approximately 0. We see that this y-value occurs when x is about 6, so we say that is will take about 6 seconds for the rocket to reach the ground.

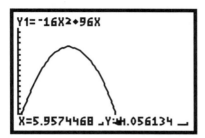

Chapter 2
Functions, Linear Equations, and Models

EVALUATING A FUNCTION

Function values can be found in several different ways on the TI-83 and the TI-83 Plus.

Section 2.1, Example 6 For $f(a) = 2a^2 - 3a + 1$, find $f(3)$ and $f(-5.1)$.

One method for finding function values involves using function notation directly. To do this, first press $\boxed{Y =}$ and enter the function on the equation-editor screen. Mentally replace a with x and $f(a)$ with Y_1. Then enter $Y_1 = 2x^2 - 3x + 1$. Now, to find $f(3)$, or $Y_1(3)$, directly first press $\boxed{\text{2nd}}$ $\boxed{\text{QUIT}}$ to go to the home screen. Then press $\boxed{\text{VARS}}$ $\boxed{\triangleright}$ 1 1 $\boxed{(}$ 3 $\boxed{)}$ $\boxed{\text{ENTER}}$. We see that $Y_1(3) = 10$, or $f(3) = 10$.

To find $f(-5.1)$, or $Y_1(-5.1)$, we can repeat the previous procedure using -5.1 in place of 3, or we can edit the previous entry. To edit, copy the entry $Y_1(3)$ to the home screen by pressing $\boxed{\text{2nd}}$ $\boxed{\text{ENTRY}}$. (ENTRY is the second operation associated with the $\boxed{\text{ENTER}}$ key.) Now replace 3 with -5.1 by first pressing $\boxed{\triangleleft}$ $\boxed{\triangleleft}$ to position the cursor over the 3. Then press $\boxed{(-)}$ to overwrite the 3 with the negative symbol. To insert 5.1 after this symbol press $\boxed{\text{2nd}}$ $\boxed{\text{INS}}$ 5 $\boxed{.}$ 1. (INS, for "insert," is the second operation associated with the $\boxed{\text{DEL}}$ key.) Finally press $\boxed{\text{ENTER}}$ to find that $Y_1(-5.1) = 68.32$, or $f(-5.1) = 68.32$.

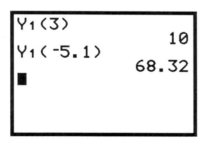

Another way to calculate a function value after the function has been entered on the equation-editor screen involves storing the input value in the calculator's memory. To find $f(3)$ for the function entered as Y_1 in this example, for instance, we can store 3 as the variable X by pressing 3 $\boxed{\text{STO} \triangleright}$ $\boxed{\text{X, T, }\Theta\text{, } n}$ $\boxed{\text{ENTER}}$. Then select Y_1 by pressing $\boxed{\text{VARS}}$ $\boxed{\triangleright}$ 1 1. Finally press $\boxed{\text{ENTER}}$ to find the value of Y_1 when $X = 3$.

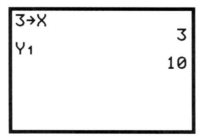

This computation can also be performed in a single step by pressing 3 $\boxed{\text{STO} \triangleright}$ $\boxed{\text{X, T, } \Theta\text{, } n}$ $\boxed{\text{ALPHA}}$ $\boxed{:}$ $\boxed{\text{VARS}}$ $\boxed{\triangleright}$ 1 1 $\boxed{\text{ENTER}}$. (The $\boxed{\text{ALPHA}}$ key is the green key below the yellow $\boxed{\text{2nd}}$ key in the left-hand column of the keypad. The symbol : is the ALPHA operation associated with the $\boxed{.}$ key.)

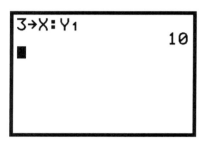

We can also find function values from the graph of the function.

Section 2.1, Example 7 Find $g(2)$ for $g(x) = 2x - 5$.

First press $\boxed{\text{Y} =}$ to go to the equation editor screen and then clear any entries that are present. Also be sure that the Stat Plots are turned off. (See page 8 of this manual for instructions for clearing equations and turning off Stat Plots.) Now enter $Y_1 = 2x - 5$ and press $\boxed{\text{ZOOM}}$ 6 to graph this function in the standard viewing window. We will use the Value feature from the CALC menu to find the value of Y_1 when $x = 2$. This is $g(2)$. Press $\boxed{\text{2nd}}$ $\boxed{\text{CALC}}$ 1 to select Value. (CALC is the second operation associated with the $\boxed{\text{TRACE}}$ key in the top row of the keypad.) Now you must supply the value of x as indicated by the blinking cursor at the bottom of the screen beside X =. Press 2 $\boxed{\text{ENTER}}$. We now see X = 2, Y = −1 at the bottom of the screen, so $g(2) = -1$.

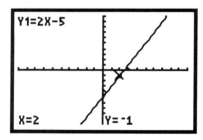

When using the Value feature, note that the x-value entered must be in the viewing window. That is, x must be a number between Xmin and Xmax.

SOLVING EQUATIONS GRAPHICALLY

We can use the Intersect feature from the CALC menu to solve equations.

Section 2.2, Example 3 Solve using a graphing calculator: $-\dfrac{3}{4}x + 6 = 2x - 1$.

On the equation editor screen, clear any existing entries and then enter $Y_1 = -(3/4)x + 6$ and $Y_2 = 2x - 1$. Although the parentheses in Y_1 are not necessary, they make the equation easier to read on the equation-editor screen. Press $\boxed{\text{ZOOM}}$ 6 to graph these equations in the standard viewing window. The solution of the equation $-\dfrac{3}{4}x + 6 = 2x - 1$ is the first coordinate of the point of intersection of these graphs. To use the Intersect feature to find this point, first press $\boxed{\text{2nd}}$ $\boxed{\text{CALC}}$ 5 to select Intersect from the CALC menu. The query "First curve?" appears at the bottom of the screen. The blinking cursor is positioned on the graph of Y_1. This is indicated by the notation $Y_1 = -\dfrac{3}{4}x + 6$ in the upper left-hand corner of the screen. Press $\boxed{\text{ENTER}}$ to indicate that this is the first curve involved in the intersection. Next the query "Second curve?" appears at the bottom of the screen. The blinking cursor is now positioned on the graph of Y_2 and the notation $Y_2 = 2x - 1$ should appear in the top left-hand corner of the screen. Press $\boxed{\text{ENTER}}$ to indicate that this is the second curve. We identify the curves for the calculator since we could have as many as ten graphs on the screen at once. After we identify the second curve, the query "Guess?" appears at the bottom of the screen. Use the right and left arrow keys to move the blinking cursor close to the point of intersection of the graphs. This provides the calculator with a guess as to the coordinates of this point. We do this since some pairs of curves can have more than one point of intersection. When the cursor is positioned, press $\boxed{\text{ENTER}}$ a third time. Now the coordinates of the point of intersection appear at the bottom of the screen.

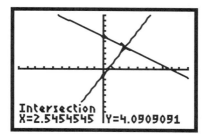

We see that $x = 2.5454545$, so the solution of the equation is 2.5454545.

We can check the solution by evaluating both sides of the equation $-\dfrac{3}{4}x + 6 = 2x - 1$ for this value of x. The first coordinate of the point of intersection has automatically been stored as X in the calculator, so we evaluate Y_1 and Y_2 for this value of X. First press $\boxed{\text{2nd}}$ $\boxed{\text{QUIT}}$ to go to the home screen. Then to evaluate Y_1 press $\boxed{\text{VARS}}$ $\boxed{\triangleright}$ 1 1 $\boxed{\text{ENTER}}$. To evaluate Y_2 press $\boxed{\text{VARS}}$ $\boxed{\triangleright}$ 1 2 $\boxed{\text{ENTER}}$. We see that Y_1 and Y_2 have the same value when X = 2.5454545, so the solution checks.

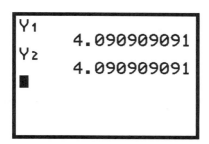

Note that although the procedure above verifies that 2.5454545 is the solution, it is actually an approximation of the solution. To find the exact solution we can solve the equation algebraically.

SOLVING FOR Y

The TI-83 and the TI-83 Plus graph only functions, so an equation must be solved for the dependent variable before it can be entered into the calculator.

Section 2.3, Example 8 Graph $3x - 4y = 2y + 7$.

We must first use our formula-solving skills to solve this equation for y. We get $y = \dfrac{-3x + 7}{-6}$. Since $y = \dfrac{-3x + 7}{-6}$ is equivalent to $3x - 4y = 2y + 7$, the graphs of these equations will be the same. Thus, we can enter the equation $Y_1 = (-3x + 7)/(-6)$ on the equation-editor screen. Note that, although the parentheses in the denominator are not necessary, they make the equation easier to read on the equation-editor screen. We graph the equation in the standard viewing window.

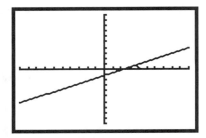

SQUARING THE VIEWING WINDOW

Section 2.5, Example 8 Determine whether the lines given by the equations $3x - y = 7$ and $x + 3y = 1$ are perpendicular, and check by graphing.

In the text each equation is solved for y in order to determine the slopes of the lines. We have $y = 3x - 7$ and $y = -\dfrac{1}{3}x + \dfrac{1}{3}$. Since $3\left(-\dfrac{1}{3}\right) = -1$, we know that the lines are perpendicular. To check this, we graph $Y_1 = 3x - 7$ and $Y_2 = -\dfrac{1}{3}x + \dfrac{1}{3}$. The graphs are shown on the right below in the standard viewing window.

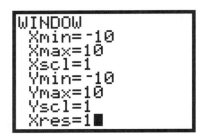
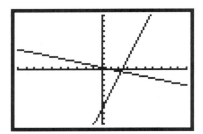

Note that the graphs do not appear to be perpendicular. This is due to the fact that, in the standard window, the distance between tick marks on the y-axis is about 2/3 the distance between tick marks on the x-axis. It is often desirable to choose window dimensions for which these distances are the same, creating a "square" window. On the TI-83 and TI-83 Plus, any window in which the ratio of the length of the y-axis to the length of the x-axis is 2/3 will produce this effect.

This can be accomplished by selecting dimensions for which Ymax $-$ Ymin $= \dfrac{2}{3}$(Xmax $-$ Xmin). For example, the windows $[-12, 12, -8, 8]$ and $[-6, 6, -4, 4]$ are square. When we change the window dimensions to $[-12, 12, -8, 8]$ and press $\boxed{\text{GRAPH}}$, the graphs now appear to be perpendicular as shown on the right below. Instead of entering window dimensions, we could also press

ZOOM 5 and the calculator will select a square window.

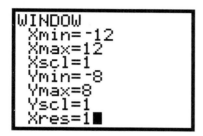 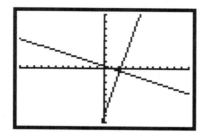

LINEAR REGRESSION

We can use the Linear Regression feature in the STAT CALC menu to fit a linear equation to a set of data.

Section 2.6, Example 5 The amount of paper recovered in the United States for various years is shown in the following table.

Years	Amount of Paper Recovered (in millions of tons)
1988	26.2
1990	29.1
1992	34.0
1994	39.7
1996	43.1
1998	45.1
2000	49.4

(a) Fit a linear function to the data.

(b) Graph the function and use it to estimate the amount of paper that will be recovered in 2003.

(a) Press STAT 1 or STAT ENTER to display the STAT lists. Clear any data previously entered in the lists. Then enter the data with the number of years since 1988 in L_1 and the number of millions of tons of paper recovered in L_2. (See page 10 of this manual for the procedure to follow to do this.)

L1	L2	L3	3
0	26.2	▬▬▬▬	
2	29.1		
4	34		
6	39.7		
8	43.1		
10	45.1		
12	49.4		

L3(1)=

Now press Y = to go to the equation-editor screen and clear any equations that are currently entered. (See page 8 of this manual.) If you wish, instead of clearing an equation, you can deselect it. To do this, position the cursor over the = sign and press ENTER . Note that the = sign is no longer highlighted, indicating that the equation has been deselected. The graph of an equation that has been deselected will not appear when $\boxed{\text{GRAPH}}$ is pressed. A deselected equation can be selected again by positioning the cursor over the = sign and pressing $\boxed{\text{ENTER}}$. Note that the = sign is once again highlighted.

Now use the graphing calculator's linear regression feature to fit a linear equation to the data. Press $\boxed{\text{STAT}}$ $\boxed{\triangleright}$ 4 $\boxed{\text{ENTER}}$ to select LinReg($ax + b$) from the STAT CALC menu and to display the coefficients a and b of the regression equation $y = ax + b$. We see that the regression equation is $y = 1.976785714x + 26.225$.

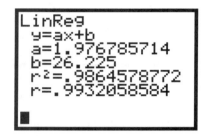

If the diagnostics have been turned on in your calculator, values for r^2 and r will also be displayed. These numbers indicate how well the regression line fits the data. For the remainder of this manual, regression will be done with the diagnostics turned off.

If you wish to select DiagnosticOn mode, press $\boxed{\text{2nd}}$ $\boxed{\text{CATALOG}}$ and use $\boxed{\triangledown}$ to position the triangular selection cursor beside DiagnosticOn. To alleviate the tedium of scrolling through many items to reach DiagnosticOn, press $\boxed{\text{D}}$ after pressing $\boxed{\text{2nd}}$ $\boxed{\text{CATALOG}}$ to move quickly to the first catalog item that begins with the letter D. (D is the ALPHA operation associated with the $\boxed{x^{-1}}$ key.) Then use $\boxed{\triangledown}$ to scroll to DiagnosticOn. Note that it is not necessary to press $\boxed{\text{ALPHA}}$ before $\boxed{\text{D}}$ when the catalog is displayed. Press $\boxed{\text{ENTER}}$ to paste this instruction to the home screen and then press $\boxed{\text{ENTER}}$ a second time to set the mode. To select DiagnosticOff mode, press $\boxed{\text{2nd}}$ $\boxed{\text{CATALOG}}$, position the selection cursor beside DiagnosticOff, press $\boxed{\text{ENTER}}$ to paste this instruction to the home screen, and then press $\boxed{\text{ENTER}}$ again to set this mode.

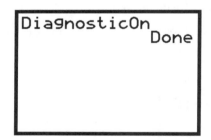
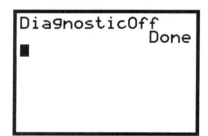

Immediately after the regression equation is found it can be copied to the equation-editor screen as Y_1. Note that any previous entry in Y_1 must have been cleared rather than deselected. Press $\boxed{Y=}$ and position the cursor beside Y_1. Then press $\boxed{\text{VARS}}$ 5 $\boxed{\triangleright}$ $\boxed{\triangleright}$ 1. These keystrokes select Statistics from the VARS menu, then select the EQ (Equation) submenu, and finally select the RegEq (Regression Equation) from this submenu.

Before the regression equation is found, it is possible to select a *y*-variable to which it will be stored on the equation editor screen. After the data have been stored in the lists and the equation previously entered as Y_1 has been cleared, press ⟨STAT⟩ ⟨▷⟩ 4 ⟨VARS⟩ ⟨▷⟩ 1 1 ⟨ENTER⟩. The coefficients of the regression equation will be displayed on the home screen, and the regression equation will also be stored as Y_1 on the equation-editor screen.

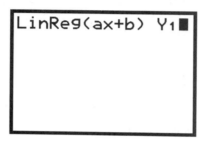

(b) Now we will graph the regression equation. In order to see the data points along with the graph of the equation we will turn on and define a Stat Plot. To do this, first press ⟨2nd⟩ ⟨STATPLOT⟩ to go to the STAT PLOTS screen. Press ⟨ENTER⟩ to select Plot 1 and then position the cursor over On and press ⟨ENTER⟩ to turn on Plot 1. Next select the scatter diagram for Type, L_1 for Xlist, L_2 for Ylist, and the box for the Mark as shown below. (See page 10 of this manual for instructions.)

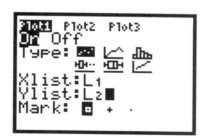

To select the dimensions of the viewing window notice that the years in the table range from 0 to 12 and the number of millions of tons of paper ranges from 26.2 to 49.4. We want to select dimensions that will include all of these values. One good choice is [0, 15, 0, 60], Yscl = 10. Enter these dimensions in the WINDOW screen.

Once the equation has been entered on the equation-editor screen as described above, press ⟨GRAPH⟩ to graph the regression line on the same axes as the data.

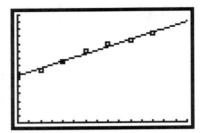

To estimate the amount of paper that will be recovered in 2003, evaluate the regression equation for $x = 15$. (2003 is 15 years after 1988.) Use any of the methods for evaluating a function presented earlier in this chapter. (See pages 15 and 169.) We will use the Value feature from the CALC menu.

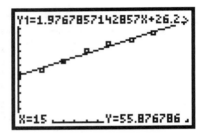

When $x = 15, y \approx 55.9$, so we estimate that about 55.9 million tons of paper will be recovered in 2003.

Chapter 3
Systems of Equations and Problem Solving

SOLVING SYSTEMS OF EQUATIONS GRAPHICALLY

We can use the Intersect feature from the CALC menu on the TI-83 and the TI-83 Plus to solve a system of two equations in two variables.

Section 3.1, Example 4(a) Solve graphically:

$$y - x = 1,$$

$$y + x = 3.$$

We graph the equations in the same viewing window and then find the coordinates of the point of intersection. Remember that equations must be entered in "$y =$" form on the equation-editor screen, so we solve both equations for y. We have $y = x + 1$ and $y = -x + 3$. Enter these equations, graph them in the standard viewing window, and find their point of intersection as described on page 17 of this manual. We see that the solution of the system of equations is $(1, 2)$.

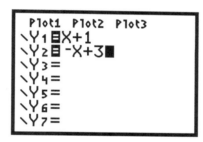
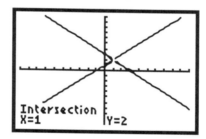

MODELS

Sometimes we model two situations with linear equations and then want to find the point of intersection of their graphs.

Section 3.1, Example 6 (d), (e) The numbers of U. S. travelers to Canada and to Europe are listed in the following table.

Year	U. S. Travelers to Canada (in millions)	U. S. Travelers to Europe (in millions)
1992	11.8	7.1
1994	12.5	8.2
1996	12.9	8.7
1998	14.9	11.1
2000	15.1	13.4

(d) Use linear regression to find two linear equations that can be used to estimate the number of U. S. travelers to Canada and Europe, in millions, x years after 1990.

(e) Use the equations found in part (d) to estimate the year in which the number of U. S. travelers to Europe will be the same as the number of U. S. travelers to Canada.

(d) Enter the data in STAT lists as described on pages 9 and 10 of this manual. We will express the years as the number of years after 1990 (in other words, 1990 is year 0) and enter them in L_1. Then enter the number of travelers to Canada, in millions, in L_2 and the number of travelers to Europe, in millions, in L_3.

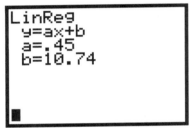

Now use linear regression to fit a linear function to the data in L_1 and L_2. The function should also be copied to the equation editor screen. We will copy it as Y_1. See pages 20 and 21 of this manual for the procedure to follow. We get $y_1 = 0.45x + 10.74$.

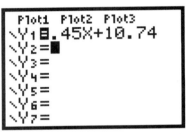

Next we fit a linear function to the data in L_1 and L_3. When combinations of lists other than L_1 and L_2 are used, the names of the lists must be entered after the linear regression command. To use L_1 and L_3, press $\boxed{\text{STAT}}$ $\boxed{\triangleright}$ $\boxed{4}$ $\boxed{\text{2nd}}$ $\boxed{L_1}$ $\boxed{,}$ $\boxed{\text{2nd}}$ $\boxed{L_3}$. (L_1 and L_3 are the second operations associated with the 1 and 3 numeric keys, respectively.) We will also copy this function to the equation-editor screen as Y_2. Note that this can be accomplished immediately after the regression equation is found by pressing $\boxed{Y =}$, positioning the cursor beside "$Y_2 =$", clearing the existing entry if one exists, and then pressing $\boxed{\text{VARS}}$ $\boxed{5}$ $\boxed{\triangleright}$ $\boxed{\triangleright}$ $\boxed{1}$. It can also be done before the regression equation is found by pressing $\boxed{,}$ $\boxed{\text{VARS}}$ $\boxed{\triangleright}$ $\boxed{1}$ $\boxed{2}$ immediately after $\boxed{L_3}$ in the sequence of keystrokes above.

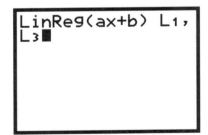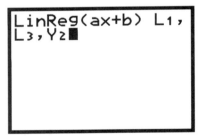

Press $\boxed{\text{ENTER}}$ to see the coefficients of the regression equation. We get $y = 0.775x + 5.05$.

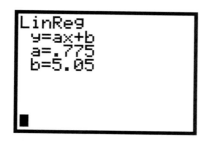 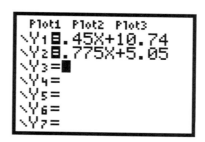

(e) To estimate the year in which the number of travelers to Europe will be the same as the number of travelers to Canada, we solve the system of equations

$$y = 0.45x + 10.74,$$

$$y = 0.775x + 5.05.$$

We graph the equations in the same viewing window and then use the Intersect feature to find their point of intersection. Through a trial-and-error process we find that $[0, 25, 0, 25]$, Xscl $= 5$, Yscl $= 5$, provides a good window in which to see this point.

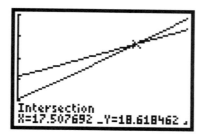

We see that the solution of the system of equations is approximately $(17.51, 18.62)$, so the number of U. S. travelers to Europe will be the same as the number of U. S. travelers to Canada about 17.5 years after 1990, or in 2008.

ELIMINATION USING MATRICES

Matrices with up to 99 rows or columns can be entered on the TI-83 and TI-83 Plus. As many as ten matrices can be entered at one time. The row-equivalent operations necessary to write a matrix in row-echelon or reduced row-echelon form can be performed on the calculator, or we can go directly to reduced row-echelon form with a single command. We will illustrate the direct approach.

Section 3.6, Example 4 Solve the following system using a graphing calculator:

$$2x + 5y - 8z = 7,$$
$$3x + 4y - 3z = 8,$$
$$5y - 2x = 9.$$

First we rewrite the third equation in the form $ax + by + cz = d$:

$$2x + 5y - 8z = 7,$$
$$3x + 4y - 3z = 8,$$
$$-2x + 5y \quad\quad = 9.$$

Then we enter the coefficient matrix

$$\begin{bmatrix} 2 & 5 & -8 & 7 \\ 3 & 4 & -3 & 8 \\ -2 & 5 & 0 & 9 \end{bmatrix}$$

in the calculator. On the TI-83 press $\boxed{\text{MATRX}}$ $\boxed{\triangleright}$ $\boxed{\triangleright}$ to display the MATRIX EDIT menu. On the TI-83 Plus press $\boxed{\text{2nd}}$ $\boxed{\text{MATRX}}$ $\boxed{\triangleright}$ $\boxed{\triangleright}$. (MATRX is the second operation associated with the $\boxed{x^{-1}}$ key on the TI-83 Plus.) Then select the matrix to be defined. We will select matrix [**A**] by pressing 1 or $\boxed{\text{ENTER}}$. Now the MATRIX EDIT screen appears. The dimensions of the matrix are displayed on the top line of this screen, with the cursor on the row dimension. Enter the dimensions of the coefficient matrix, 3 x 4, by pressing 3 $\boxed{\text{ENTER}}$ 4 $\boxed{\text{ENTER}}$. Now the cursor moves to the element in the first row and first column of the matrix. Enter the elements of the first row by pressing 2 $\boxed{\text{ENTER}}$ 5 $\boxed{\text{ENTER}}$ $\boxed{(-)}$ 8 $\boxed{\text{ENTER}}$ 7 $\boxed{\text{ENTER}}$. The cursor moves to the element in the second row and first column of the matrix. Enter the elements of the second and third rows of the augmented matrix by typing each in turn followed by $\boxed{\text{ENTER}}$ as above. Note that the screen only displays three columns of the matrix. The arrow keys can be used to move the cursor to any element at any time.

Matrix operations are found on the MATRIX MATH menu and are performed on the home screen. Press $\boxed{\text{2nd}}$ $\boxed{\text{QUIT}}$ to leave the matrix editor and go to the home screen. Then, on the TI-83, press $\boxed{\text{MATRX}}$ $\boxed{\triangleright}$ to access the MATRIX MATH menu. On the TI-83 Plus press $\boxed{\text{2nd}}$ $\boxed{\text{MATRX}}$ $\boxed{\triangleright}$. The reduced row-echelon form command is item B on this menu. Copy it to the home screen by using the $\boxed{\triangledown}$ key to scroll down until "B" is highlighted and then press $\boxed{\text{ENTER}}$ or by simply pressing $\boxed{\text{ALPHA}}$ B. (We could also use the $\boxed{\triangle}$ key to scroll up to "B" and then press $\boxed{\text{ENTER}}$.) We see the command "rref(" on the home screen.

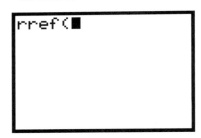

Since we want to find reduced row-echelon form for matrix [**A**], we enter [**A**] on the TI-83 by pressing $\boxed{\text{MATRX}}$ $\boxed{\text{ENTER}}$ $\boxed{)}$ or $\boxed{\text{MATRX}}$ 1 $\boxed{)}$. On the TI-83 Plus press $\boxed{\text{2nd}}$ $\boxed{\text{MATRX}}$ $\boxed{\text{ENTER}}$ $\boxed{)}$ or $\boxed{\text{2nd}}$ $\boxed{\text{MATRX}}$ 1 $\boxed{)}$. On either calculator we also press $\boxed{\text{MATH}}$ 1 or $\boxed{\text{MATH}}$ $\boxed{\text{ENTER}}$ to see the elements of the reduced row-echelon form of the matrix in fraction form. Finally press $\boxed{\text{ENTER}}$ to see the reduced row-echelon matrix. In the right-hand column we see that the solution of the system of equations is $\left(\frac{1}{2}, 2, \frac{1}{2}\right)$.

```
rref([A])▶Frac
   [[1 0 0 1/2]
    [0 1 0 2  ]
    [0 0 1 1/2]]
■
```

Chapter 4
Inequalities and Problem Solving

GRAPHICAL SOLUTIONS OF INEQUALITIES

Solving inequalities graphically involves first finding a point of intersection.

Section 4.1, Example 4 Solve graphically: $16 - 7x \geq 10x - 4$.

Graph $y_1 = 16 - 7x$ and $y_2 = 10x - 4$ in the window $[-5, 5, -5, 15]$ and find the first coordinate of their point of intersection. It is approximately 1.1764706.

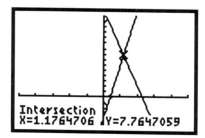

Observe that y_1 (on the graph that slants down from left to right) is greater than y_2 (on the graph that slants up from left to right) to the left of the point of intersection and $y_1 < y_2$ to the right of this point. Thus, the solution set will consist of all x-values to the left of 1.1764706 and also the value 1.1764706 itself since the inequality symbol is $\geq$, or $(-\infty, 1.1764706]$.

Another method for solving inequalities on a graphing calculator makes use of the $\boxed{\text{VARS}}$ and $\boxed{\text{TEST}}$ keys. To solve the inequality above this way, we begin as before by finding the first coordinate of the point of intersection of y_1 and y_2. Then return to the equation-editor screen and enter $y_3 = y_1 \geq y_2$ by positioning the cursor beside $Y_3 =$ and pressing $\boxed{\text{VARS}}$ $\boxed{\triangleright}$ 1 1 $\boxed{\text{2nd}}$ $\boxed{\text{TEST}}$ 4 $\boxed{\text{VARS}}$ $\boxed{\triangleright}$ 1 2. (TEST is the second operation associated with the $\boxed{\text{MATH}}$ key.) The first four keystrokes enter Y_1, the next three display the TEST menu and paste the symbol "$\geq$" from that menu to the equation-editor screen, and the last four enter Y_2 after $\geq$.

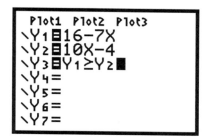

The value of y_3 will be 1 where $y_1 \geq y_2$ is true, and it will be 0 where $y_1 \geq y_2$ is false. Press $\boxed{\text{GRAPH}}$ to see the graphs of y_1, y_2, and y_3. We use the same window as above.

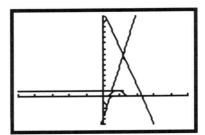

The solution set of $y_1 \geq y_2$ is displayed as an interval shown by a horizontal line 1 unit above the x-axis. The endpoint of this interval corresponds to the first coordinate of the point of intersection of y_1 and y_2. Thus, we see again that the solution set of the original inequality is approximately $(-\infty, 1.1764706]$.

INEQUALITIES IN TWO VARIABLES

The solution set of an inequality in two variables can be graphed on the TI-83 and the TI-83 Plus.

Section 4.4, Example 4 Use a graphing calculator to graph the inequality $8x + 3y > 24$.

First we write the related equation, $8x + 3y = 24$, and solve it for y. We get $y = -\frac{8}{3}x + 8$. We will enter this as Y$_1$. Press $\boxed{Y =}$ to go to the equation-editor screen. If there is currently an entry for Y$_1$, clear it. Also clear or deselect any other equations that are entered. Now enter $y_1 = (-8/3)x + 8$. Since the inequality states that $8x + 3y > 24$, or y is *greater than* $-\frac{8}{3}x + 8$, we want to shade the half-plane above the graph of y_1. To do this, move the cursor to the GraphStyle icon to the left of Y$_1$ and press $\boxed{\text{ENTER}}$ repeatedly until the symbol indicating the "shade above" GraphStyle appears. If the "line" GraphStyle was previously selected, the "Shade above" icon will appear after $\boxed{\text{ENTER}}$ is pressed two times. (To shade below a line we would press $\boxed{\text{ENTER}}$ until the "shade below" GraphStyle symbol appears.) Then press $\boxed{\text{ZOOM}}$ 6 to see the graph of the inequality in the standard viewing window.

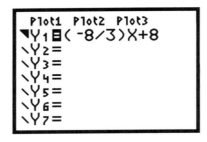
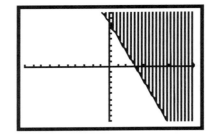

Note that when the "shade above" GraphStyle is selected it is not also possible to select the dotted GraphStyle so we must keep in mind the fact that the line $y = -\frac{8}{3}x + 8$ is not included in the graph of the inequality. If you graphed this inequality by hand, you would draw a dashed line.

SYSTEMS OF LINEAR INEQUALITIES

We can graph systems of inequalities by shading the solution set of each inequality in the system with a different pattern. When the "shade above" or "shade below" GraphStyle options are selected the calculator rotates through four shading patterns. Vertical lines shade the first function, horizontal lines the second, negatively sloping diagonal lines the third, and positively sloping diagonal lines the fourth. These patterns repeat if more than four functions are graphed.

Section 4.4, Example 8 Graph the system

$$x + y \leq 4,$$

$$x - y < 4.$$

First graph the equation $x + y = 4$, entering it in the form $y = -x + 4$. We determine that the solution set of $x + y \leq 4$ consists of all points on or below the line $x + y = 4$, or $y = -x + 4$, so we select the "shade below" GraphStyle for this function. Next graph $x - y = 4$, entering it in the form $y = x - 4$. The solution set of $x - y < 4$ is all points above the line $x - y = 4$, or $y = x - 4$, so for this function we choose the "shade above" GraphStyle. (See Example 4 above for instructions on selecting GraphStyle icons.) Now press $\boxed{\text{ZOOM}}$ 6 to display the solution sets of each inequality in the system and the region where they overlap in the standard viewing window. The region of overlap is the solution set of the system of inequalities. Keep in mine that the line $x + y = 4$, or $y = -x + 4$, is part of the solution set while $x - y = 4$, or $y = x - 4$, is not.

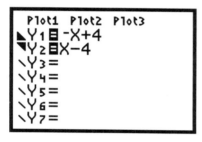
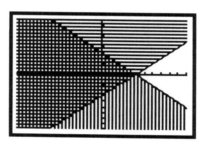

Chapter 5
Polynomials and Polynomial Functions

EVALUATING A POLYNOMIAL FUNCTION

We can use a table set in Ask mode to evaluate a polynomial function.

Section 5.1, Example 4 Find $P(-5)$ for the polynomial function given by $P(x) = -x^2 + 4x - 1$.

To use a table to find this function value, first enter $Y_1 = -x^2 + 4x - 1$ on the equation-editor screen. Then press $\boxed{\text{2nd}}$ $\boxed{\text{TblSet}}$ to display the table set-up screen. (TblSet is the second operation associated with the $\boxed{\text{WINDOW}}$ key.) To set up a table in which you choose the x-values that are entered, set "Indpnt" to "Ask" by positioning the cursor over "Ask" and pressing $\boxed{\text{ENTER}}$. "Depend" should be set to "Auto." In Ask mode the calculator disregards the setting of TblStart and ΔTbl.

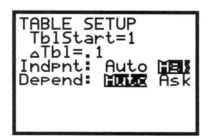

Now press $\boxed{\text{2nd}}$ $\boxed{\text{TABLE}}$ to view the table. (TABLE is the second operation associated with the $\boxed{\text{GRAPH}}$ key.) Values for x can be entered in the X-column of the table and the corresponding y-values will be displayed in the Y_1-column. To enter -5 for x, press $\boxed{(-)}$ 5 $\boxed{\text{ENTER}}$. We see that $P(-5) = -46$.

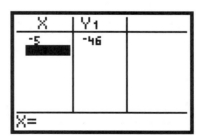

CHECKING OPERATIONS ON POLYNOMIALS

A graphing calculator can be used to check operations on polynomials.

Section 5.1, Example 9 Add: $(-3x^3 + 2x - 4) + (4x^3 + 3x^2 + 2)$.

This addition is carried out in the text, and the result is $x^3 + 3x^2 + 2x - 2$. There are several ways in which we can use a graphing calculator to check this result. One of these is to compare the graphs of $Y_1 = (-3x^3 + 2x - 4) + (4x^3 + 3x^2 + 2)$ and

$Y_2 = x^3 + 3x^2 + 2x - 2$. This is most easily done when different graph styles are used for the graphs.

Seven graph styles can be selected on the equation-editor screen of the TI-83 and the TI-83 Plus. The **path graph style** can be used, along with the line style, to determine whether graphs coincide. To use graphs to check the addition in Example 9, first press $\boxed{\text{MODE}}$ to determine whether Sequential mode is selected. If it is not, position the blinking cursor over Sequential and then press $\boxed{\text{ENTER}}$. Next, on the Y = screen, enter $Y_1 = (-3x^3 + 2x - 4) + (4x^3 + 3x^2 + 2)$ and $Y_2 = x^3 + 3x^2 + 2x - 2$. We will select the line graph style for Y_1 and the path style for Y_2. To select these graph styles use $\boxed{\triangleleft}$ to position the cursor over the icon to the left of the equation and press $\boxed{\text{ENTER}}$ repeatedly until the desired style icon appears as shown on the right below.

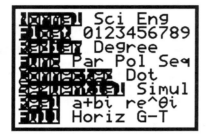
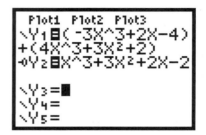

The calculator will graph Y_1 first as a solid line. Then Y_2 will be graphed as the circular cursor traces the leading edge of the graph, allowing us to determine visually whether the graphs coincide. In this case, the graphs appear to coincide, so the factorization is probably correct.

We can also check the addition by **subtracting** the result from the original sum. With Y_1 and Y_2 entered as described above, position the cursor beside "$Y_3 =$" and use the Y-VARS menu to enter $Y_3 = Y_1 - Y_2$ by pressing $\boxed{\text{VARS}}$ $\boxed{\triangleright}$ 1 1 $\boxed{(-)}$ $\boxed{\text{VARS}}$ $\boxed{\triangleright}$ 1 2. If the expressions for Y_1 and Y_2 are equivalent, the graph of Y_3 will be $y = 0$, or the x-axis. Since we are interested only in the values of Y_3, deselect Y_1 and Y_2 as described on page 19 of this manual and select the path graph style for Y_3 as described above.

Now press $\boxed{\text{GRAPH}}$ and determine if the graph of Y_3 is traced over the x-axis. Since it is, the sum is correct.

We can use a table of values to **compare values** of Y_1 and Y_2. If the expressions for Y_1 and Y_2 are the same for each given x-value, the result checks. If you deselected Y_1 and Y_2 to check the sum using subtraction as described above, select them again now. Then look at a table set in Auto mode. Since the values of Y_1 and Y_2 are the same for each given x-value, the result checks. Scrolling through the table to look at additional values makes this conclusion more certain.

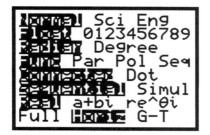

We can also check the sum in Example 9 using a **horizontal split-screen**. The top half of the screen displays the graph and, in this case, we will use the bottom half to display a table of values.

First enter Y_1 and Y_2 as described above. Then, to select the horizontal split-screen option, press $\boxed{\text{MODE}}$ to access the Mode screen. Position the cursor over Horiz on the last line and press $\boxed{\text{ENTER}}$. Press $\boxed{\text{GRAPH}}$ to see the graph in the top half of the split screen, and press $\boxed{\text{2nd}}$ $\boxed{\text{TABLE}}$ to see two lines of the table of values for y_1 and y_2 below the graph. We show these functions graphed in the standard window. We show a table with TblStart $= -3$, ΔTbl $= 1$, and Indpnt and Depend both set on Auto. The graphs appear to coincide. In addition, as we scroll through the table, we see that the values of Y_1 and Y_2 are the same for any given x-value, so the sum is probably correct.

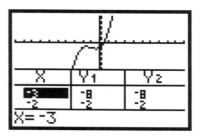

The lower half of the split screen can also display four lines of the home screen, four lines of the equation-editor screen, two rows of the Stat list editor screen, or three settings of the Window screen instead of two lines of the table. To change from the table to the home screen, press $\boxed{\text{2nd}}$ $\boxed{\text{QUIT}}$. Display the equation-editor screen by pressing $\boxed{\text{Y} =}$, the Stat list editor by pressing $\boxed{\text{STAT}}$ 1, or the Window screen by pressing $\boxed{\text{WINDOW}}$.

In order to return to a full-screen graph, table, equation-editor, Stat list editor, or window screen, return to the Mode screen and select Full.

We can also use a **vertical split screen** to check Example 9. First enter Y_1, Y_2, and Y_3 as described above and deselect Y_1 and Y_2. Then press $\boxed{\text{MODE}}$ to display the Mode screen, position the cursor over G-T on the last line, and press $\boxed{\text{ENTER}}$. Now press $\boxed{\text{GRAPH}}$ to see the graph of Y_3 on the left side of the screen and a table of values for Y_3 on the right side. As we did above, we use a table set in Auto mode with TblStart $= -3$ and ΔTbl $= 1$. Since the graph appears to be $y = 0$, or the x-axis, and all of the Y_3-values in the table are 0, we confirm that the result is correct.

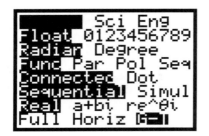 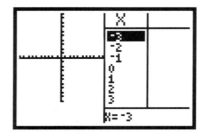

In order to return to full-screen mode, return to the Mode screen and select Full.

FINDING THE ZEROS OF A FUNCTION

We can use the Zero feature from the CALC menu to find the zeros of a function.

Section 5.3, Example 2 Find the zeros of the function given by $f(x) = x^3 - 3x^2 - 4x + 12$.

First we graph the function in a viewing window that shows the x-intercepts clearly. Through a trial-and-error process we find that $[-5, 5, -20, 20]$, Yscl $= 2$, is a god choice. We see that the function has three zeros. They appear to be about -2, 2, and 3.

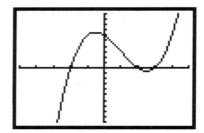

We will find the zero near -2 first. Press $\boxed{\text{2nd}}$ $\boxed{\text{CALC}}$ 2 to select the Zero feature from the CALC menu. We are prompted to select a left bound. This means that we must choose an x-value that is to the left of -2 on the x-axis. This can be done by using the left- and right-hand arrow keys to move to a point on the curve to the left of -2 or by keying in a value less than -2.

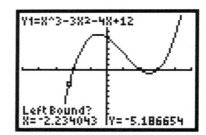

Once this is done, press $\boxed{\text{ENTER}}$. Now we are prompted to select a right bound that is to the right of -2 on the x-axis. Again, this can be done by using the arrow keys to move to a point on the curve to the right of -2 or by keying in a value greater than -2.

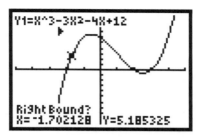

Press ENTER again. Finally we are prompted to make a guess as to the value of the zero. Move the cursor to a point close to the zero or key in a value.

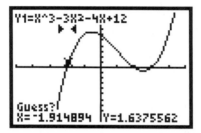

Press ENTER a third time. We see that $y = 0$ when $x = -2$, so -2 is a zero of the function f.

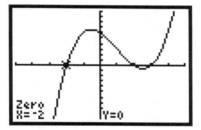

Select ZERO from the CALC menu a second time to find the zero near 2 and a third time to find the zero near 3. We see that the other two zeros are exactly 2 and 3.

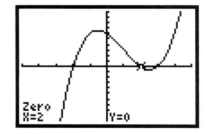
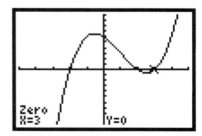

POLYNOMIAL REGRESSION

The TI-83 and TI-83 Plus have the capability to use regression to fit nonlinear polynomial equations to data.

Section 5.8, Example 4(a) The number of bachelor's degrees earned in the biological and life sciences for various years is shown in the following table. Fit a polynomial function of degree 3 (cubic) to the data.

Year	Number of Bachelor's Degrees Earned in Biological/Life Science
1971	35,743
1976	54,275
1980	46,370
1986	38,524
1990	37,204
1994	51,383
2000	63,532

First enter the data with the number of years since 1970 in L_1 and the number of bachelor's degrees earned, in thousands, in L_2. (See pages 9 and 10 of this manual for the procedure to follow.) We select cubic regression, denoted CubicReg, from the STAT CALC menu. Press $\boxed{\text{STAT}}$ $\boxed{\triangleright}$ 6 $\boxed{\text{ENTER}}$. (Note that if the data are entered in a combination of lists other than L_1 and L_2 these lists must be specified. See page 24 of this manual.) The calculator returns the coefficients for a cubic function of the form $f(x) = ax^3 + bx^2 + cx + d$. Rounding the coefficients to the nearest thousandth, we have $f(x) = 0.009x^3 - 0.371x^2 + 4.176x + 34.415$.

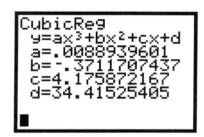

We can use methods discussed earlier in this manual to estimate and predict function values and to find the year or years in which a specific function value occurs.

Chapter 6
Rational Equations and Functions

GRAPHING IN DOT MODE

Consider the graph of the function $T(t) = \dfrac{t^2 + 5t}{2t + 5}$ in Section 6.1, Example 1. Enter $y = (x^2 + 5x)/(2x + 5)$ and graph it in the window $[-5, 5, -5, 5]$.

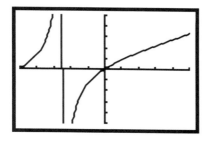

Note that a vertical line that is not part of the graph appears on the screen along with the two branches of the graph. The reason for this is discussed in the text.

This line will not appear if we change from Connected mode to Dot mode. Access the Mode screen by pressing $\boxed{\text{MODE}}$. Then move the cursor to Dot on the fifth line and press $\boxed{\text{ENTER}}$. Now press $\boxed{\text{GRAPH}}$ to see the graph of the function in Dot mode.

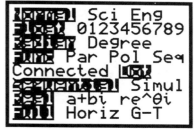 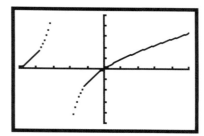

We can also select Dot mode by selecting the "dot" GraphStyle on the equation-editor screen. If the function $T(t) = \dfrac{t^2 + 5t}{2t + 5}$ is entered as $y_1 = (x^2 + 5x)/(2x + 5)$, for instance, position the cursor over the GraphStyle icon to the left of Y_1 and press $\boxed{\text{ENTER}}$ repeatedly until the "dot" icon appears. If the "line" icon was previously selected, $\boxed{\text{ENTER}}$ must be pressed six times to select the "dot" style.

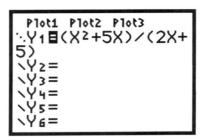

It should be noted that, when an equation is cleared on the equation-editor screen of the TI-83 or the TI-83 Plus, the GraphStyle returns to "line" (or connected mode) regardless of the mode selected on the MODE screen.

Chapter 7
Exponents and Radical Functions

RADICAL EXPRESSIONS AND RATIONAL EXPONENTS

As discussed in Section 7.2, we can enter a radical expression using radical notation or rational exponents. For example, we can enter $y = \sqrt{x-3}$ using radical notation or as $y = (x-2)^{1/2}$ or as $y = (x-3)^{0.5}$. To enter $= \sqrt{x-3}$, press $\boxed{\text{2nd}}$ $\boxed{\sqrt{}}$ $\boxed{\text{X, T, } \Theta, n}$ $\boxed{-}$ 3 $\boxed{)}$. ($\sqrt{}$ is the second operation associated with the $\boxed{x^2}$ key.) Note that the calculator supplies the left parenthesis along with the radical symbol and we add a right parenthesis after entering the radicand. To enter $y = (x-3)^{1/2}$, press $\boxed{(}$ $\boxed{\text{X, T, } \Theta, n}$ $\boxed{-}$ 3 $\boxed{)}$ $\boxed{\wedge}$ $\boxed{(}$ 1 $\boxed{\div}$ 2 $\boxed{)}$. Note that both the radicand and the rational exponent are enclosed in parentheses. To enter $y = (x-3)^{0.5}$, press $\boxed{(}$ $\boxed{\text{X, T, } \Theta, n}$ $\boxed{-}$ 3 $\boxed{)}$ $\boxed{\wedge}$ 0 $\boxed{\cdot}$ 5. When the exponent is in decimal notation it is not necessary to enclose it in parentheses.

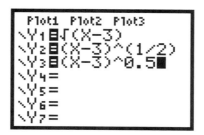

We can use either the cube root option or a rational exponent to enter a cube root. For example, to enter $y = \sqrt[3]{x+5}$ using radical notation we press $\boxed{\text{MATH}}$ 4 $\boxed{\text{X, T, } \Theta, n}$ $\boxed{+}$ 5 $\boxed{)}$. The keystrokes $\boxed{\text{MATH}}$ 4 access the MATH MATH menu and then select item 4, the cube root option, from that menu. As with the square root option, the calculator supplies a left parenthesis and we close the parentheses after entering the radicand. Using a rational exponent, we can enter $y = \sqrt[3]{x+5}$ as $y = (x+5)^{1/3}$. Press $\boxed{(}$ $\boxed{\text{X, T, } \Theta, n}$ $\boxed{+}$ 5 $\boxed{)}$ $\boxed{\wedge}$ $\boxed{(}$ 1 $\boxed{\div}$ 3 $\boxed{)}$. Since we cannot enter exact decimal notation for 1/3, we cannot use decimal notation for the exponent in this case.

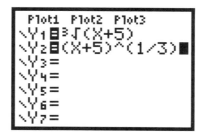

To enter $f(x) = \sqrt[4]{2x-7}$, as in Section 7.2, Example 3, we use the xth root option from the MATH MATH menu. To do this we first enter the index of the radical, 4. Then select the xth root feature and, finally, enter the radicand, $2x-7$. Press 4 $\boxed{\text{MATH}}$

5 $\boxed{(}$ 2 $\boxed{\text{X, T, }\Theta, n}$ $\boxed{-}$ 7 $\boxed{)}$. Note that the calculator does not supply a left parenthesis with this option, so we enter it ourselves. We could also enter this function as $f(x) = (2x - 7)^{1/4}$ or as $f(x) = (2x - 7)^{0.25}$.

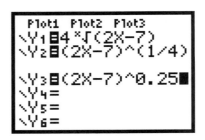

Chapter 8
Quadratic Functions and Equations

FINDING THE VERTEX

We can use a graphing calculator to find the vertex of a quadratic function. We do this by using the Maximum or Minimum feature from the CALC menu.

Section 8.7, Example 4 Use a graphing calculator to determine the vertex of the graph of the function given by $f(x) = -2x^2 + 10x - 7$.

The coefficient of x^2 is negative, so we know that the graph of the function opens down and, thus, has a maximum value. Clear or deselect any functions previously entered on the equation-editor screen. Then enter $y = -2x^2 + 10x - 7$. Choose a viewing window that shows the vertex. One good choice is $[-3, 7, -10, 10]$.

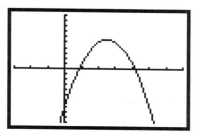

Now select the Maximum feature from the CALC menu by pressing $\boxed{\text{2nd}}$ $\boxed{\text{CALC}}$ 4. We are prompted to select a left bound for the vertex. Use the arrow keys to move the cursor to a point on the parabola to the left of the vertex or key in an x-value that is less than the x-coordinate of the vertex.

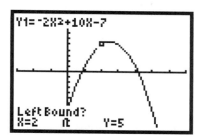

Press $\boxed{\text{ENTER}}$. Next we are prompted to select a right bound. Move the cursor to a point on the parabola to the right of the vertex or key in an x-value that is greater than the x-coordinate of the vertex.

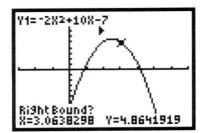

Press ENTER . We are now prompted to make a guess as to the x-coordinate of the vertex. Move the cursor close to the vertex or key in an x-value close to the x-value of the vertex.

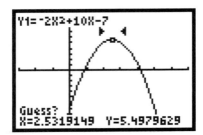

Press ENTER a third time. We see that the maximum function value is 5.5, and it occurs when x is approximately 2.5. Thus, the vertex of the graph of $f(x) = -2x^2 + 10x - 7$ is $(2.5, 5.5)$. (Note that, because of the method the calculator uses to find the maximum function value, the coordinates might not be exact and can vary slightly depending on the window chosen.)

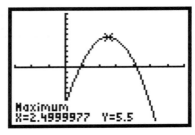

Minimum function values are found in a similar manner. Select the Minimum feature from the CALC menu by pressing 2nd CALC 3.

QUADRATIC REGRESSION

Regression can be used to fit a quadratic function to data when three or more data points are given.

Section 8.8, Example 4(c) According to the Centers for Disease Control and Prevention, the percent of high school students who reported having smoked a cigarette in the preceding 30 days declined from 1997 to 2001, after rising in the first part of the 1990s. Use the REGRESSION feature of a graphing calculator to fit a quadratic function $H(x)$ to all the given data in the following table.

Years after 1991	Percent of High School Students Who Smoked a Cigarette in the Preceding 30 Days
0	27.5
2	30.5
4	34.9
6	36.4
8	34.9
10	28.5

We enter the data in L_1 and L_2 as described on pages 9 and 10 of this manual.

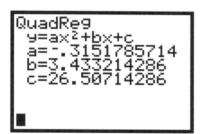

Then select QuadReg from the STAT CALC menu by pressing $\boxed{\text{STAT}}$ $\boxed{\text{CALC}}$ 5 $\boxed{\text{ENTER}}$. The calculator returns the coefficients of a quadratic function $y = ax^2 + bx + c$. From the screen below we see that we have $H(x) = -0.3151785714x^2 + 3.433214286x + 26.50714286$.

In order to use this function to perform computations it must be copied to the equation-editor screen. See pages 20 and 21 of this manual for the procedure to follow. The function can be evaluated using one of the methods on pages 15 and 16.

Chapter 9
Exponential and Logarithmic Functions

COMPOSITE FUNCTIONS

For functions y_1 and y_2, when we enter $y_1(y_2)$ on a TI-83 or TI-83 Plus we are entering the composition $y_1 \circ y_2$. The composite functions found in Section 9.1, Example 2 are checked using tables on a graphing calculator. To check that $f \circ g = \sqrt{x-1}$ when $f(x) = \sqrt{x}$ and $g(x) = x - 1$, enter $y_1 = \sqrt{x}$, $y_2 = x - 1$, $y_3 = \sqrt{x-1}$, and $y_4 = y_1(y_2)$ on the equation-editor screen. We use the VARS Y-VARS menu to enter y_4. To do this, position the cursor beside $Y_4 =$ and press $\boxed{\text{VARS}}$ $\boxed{\triangleright}$ 1 1 $\boxed{(}$ $\boxed{\text{VARS}}$ $\boxed{\triangleright}$ 1 2 $\boxed{)}$. Then compare the values of y_3 and y_4 in a table. We show a table with TblStart $= 1$, ΔTbl $= 0.5$, and Indpnt and Depend both set on Auto. Use the $\boxed{\triangleright}$ key to scroll across the table to see the Y_3- and Y_4-columns.

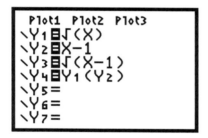

Similarly, to check that $g \circ f(x) = \sqrt{x} - 1$, also enter $y_5 = \sqrt{x} - 1$ and $y_6 = y_2(y_1)$. To enter y_6, position the cursor beside $Y_6 =$ and press $\boxed{\text{VARS}}$ $\boxed{\triangleright}$ 1 2 $\boxed{(}$ $\boxed{\text{VARS}}$ $\boxed{\triangleright}$ 1 1 $\boxed{)}$.

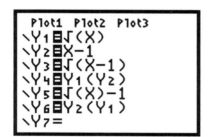

GRAPHING FUNCTIONS AND THEIR INVERSES

We can graph the inverse of a function using the DrawInv feature from the DRAW menu.

Section 9.1, Example 9(c) Graph the inverse of the function $g(x) = x^3 + 2$.

We will graph $g(x)$, $g^{-1}(x)$, and the line $y = x$ on the same screen. Press $\boxed{Y =}$ to go to the equation-editor screen and clear or deselect any existing entries. Then enter $y_1 = x^3 + 2$ and $y_2 = x$. Select a square window by pressing $\boxed{\text{ZOOM}}$ 5. Now paste the DrawInv command from the DRAW DRAW menu to the home screen by pressing $\boxed{\text{2nd}}$ $\boxed{\text{DRAW}}$ 8. Indicate that we want to draw the inverse of y_1 by pressing $\boxed{\text{VARS}}$ $\boxed{\triangleright}$ 1 1. Finally press $\boxed{\text{ENTER}}$ to see the graph of y_1^{-1} along with the graphs of y_1 and y_2. We show a window that has been squared from the standard window.

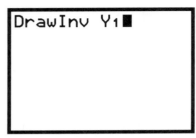
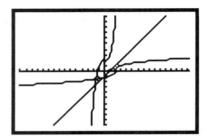

The drawing of y_1^{-1} can be cleared from the graph screen by pressing $\boxed{\text{2nd}}$ $\boxed{\text{DRAW}}$ 1 to select the ClrDraw (clear drawing) operation. If ClrDraw was not accessed from the graph screen, it must be followed by $\boxed{\text{ENTER}}$. The graph will also be cleared when another function is subsequently entered on the "Y =" screen and graphed.

GRAPHING LOGARITHMIC FUNCTIONS

Section 9.3, Example 4 Graph: $f(x) = \log \dfrac{x}{5} + 1$.

We enter $y = \log(x/5) + 1$ on the equation-editor screen by positioning the cursor beside one of the function names and pressing $\boxed{\text{LOG}}$ $\boxed{\text{X, T, }\Theta, n}$ $\boxed{\div}$ 5 $\boxed{)}$ $\boxed{+}$ 1. Note that the parentheses must be closed in the denominator of the logarithmic function. (Clear or deselect any previously entered functions.) We show the function graphed in the window $[-2, 10, -5, 5]$.

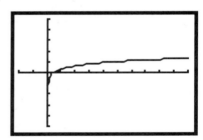

MORE ON GRAPHING

Section 9.5, Example 4 Graph: $f(x) = e^{-0.5x} + 1$.

We enter $y = e^{-0.5x} + 1$ on the equation-editor screen by positioning the cursor beside one of the function names and pressing $\boxed{\text{2nd}}$ $\boxed{e^x}$ $\boxed{(-)}$ $\boxed{.}$ 5 $\boxed{\text{X, T, }\Theta, n}$ $\boxed{)}$ $\boxed{+}$ 1. (Clear or deselect any previously entered functions.) Select a window and press $\boxed{\text{GRAPH}}$. We show the function graphed in the window $[-5, 5, -2, 10]$.

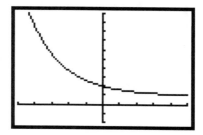

Section 9.5, Example 5(b) Graph: $f(x) = \ln(x + 3)$.

We enter $y = \ln(x + 3)$ on the equation-editor screen by positioning the cursor beside one of the function names and pressing $\boxed{\text{LN}}$ $\boxed{\text{X, T, } \Theta, n}$ $\boxed{+}$ 3 $\boxed{)}$. (Clear or deselect any previously entered functions.) Select a window and press $\boxed{\text{GRAPH}}$. We show the function graphed in the window $[-5, 10, -5, 5]$.

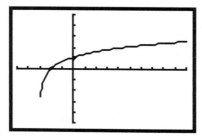

Section 9.5, Example 6 Graph: $f(x) = \log_7 x + 2$.

To use a graphing calculator we must first change the logarithmic base to e or 10. We will use e here. Recall that the change of base formula is $\log_b M = \dfrac{\log_a M}{\log_a b}$, where a and b are any logarithmic bases and M is any positive number. Let $a = e$, $b = 7$, and $M = x$ and substitute in the change-of-base formula. After clearing or deselecting previously entered functions, enter $y_1 = \dfrac{\ln x}{\ln 7} + 2$ on the equation-editor screen by positioning the cursor beside Y$_1$ = and pressing $\boxed{\text{LN}}$ $\boxed{\text{X, T, } \Theta, n}$ $\boxed{)}$ $\boxed{\div}$ $\boxed{\text{LN}}$ 7 $\boxed{)}$ $\boxed{+}$ 2. Note that the parentheses must be closed in both the numerator and the denominator.

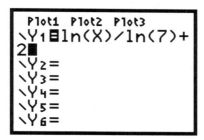

Select a viewing window and press $\boxed{\text{GRAPH}}$. We show the graph in the window $[-2, 8, -2, 5]$.

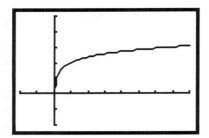

EXPONENTIAL REGRESSION

The STAT CALC menu contains an exponential regression feature.

Section 9.7, Example 9(a) In 1800, over 500,000 Tule elk inhabited the state of California. By the late 1800s, after the California Gold Rush, there were fewer than 50 elk remaining in the state. In 1978, wildlife biologists introduced a herd of 10 Tule elk into the Point Reyes National Seashore near San Francisco. By 1982, the herd had grown to 24 elk. There were 70 elk in 1986, 200 in 1996, and 500 in 2002. Use regression to fit an exponential function to the data and graph the function.

We enter the data as described on pages 9 and 10 of this manual. Let x represent the number of years since 1978.

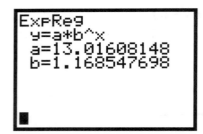

Now select ExpReg from the STAT CALC menu by pressing $\boxed{\text{STAT}}$ $\boxed{\triangleright}$ $\boxed{0}$ $\boxed{\text{ENTER}}$ and also press $\boxed{\text{VARS}}$ $\boxed{\triangleright}$ 1 1 to copy the regression equation to the "Y =" screen. The calculator returns the values of a and b for the exponential function $y = ab^x$. We have $y = 13.01608148(1.168547698)^x$. We graph the equation in the window $[-2, 40, -5, 1000]$, Xscl = 5, Yscl = 100.

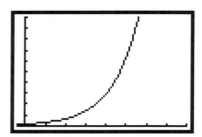

This function can be evaluated using one of the methods on pages 15 and 16.

Chapter 10
Sequences, Series, and the Binomial Theorem

SEQUENCE MODE

To enter a sequence in a graphing calculator, first select Seq (Sequence) mode.

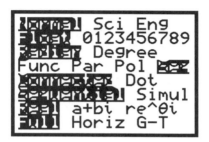

When the $\boxed{\text{X, T, } \Theta, n}$ key is pressed in Sequence mode, the variable that appears is n instead of x. In addition, the function names that appear on the equation-editor screen when $\boxed{\text{Y} =}$ is pressed are u, v, and w rather than Y_1, Y_2, and so on.

Section 10.1, Example 1 Find the first four terms and the 13th term of the sequence for which the general term is given by $a_n = (-1)^n n^2$.

After selecting Sequence mode, press $\boxed{\text{Y} =}$ to go to the sequence-editor screen. The minimum value of n in this sequence is 1, so we set $n\text{Min} = 1$. Then we enter the general term of the sequence beside "$u(n) =$" by pressing $\boxed{(}$ $\boxed{(-)}$ $\boxed{1}$ $\boxed{)}$ $\boxed{\wedge}$ $\boxed{\text{X, T, } \Theta, n}$ $\boxed{\times}$ $\boxed{\text{X, T, } \Theta, n}$ $\boxed{x^2}$.

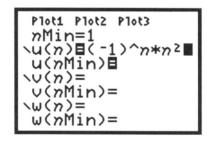

Now set up a table with Indpnt set to Ask. (See page 33 of this manual.) To see the first four terms and the 13th term of the sequence enter 1, 2, 3, 4, and 13 for n in the table.

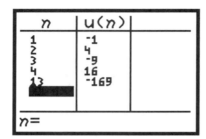

THE SEQUENCE FEATURE

The Sequence feature of the TI-83 and the TI-83 Plus writes the terms of a sequence as a list. This feature can be used even if the calculator is not in Sequence mode.

Section 10.1, Example 2 Use a graphing calculator to find the first five terms of the sequence for which the general term is given by $a_n = n/(n+1)^2$.

We will copy the Sequence feature from the LIST OPS menu to the home screen by pressing $\boxed{\text{2nd}}$ $\boxed{\text{LIST}}$ $\boxed{\triangleright}$ 5. (LIST is the second operation associated with the $\boxed{\text{STAT}}$ key.) Now enter the general term of the sequence, the variable, and the values of the variable for the first and last terms we wish to calculate, all separated by commas. Press $\boxed{\text{X, T, }\Theta, n}$ $\boxed{\div}$ $\boxed{(}$ $\boxed{\text{X, T, }\Theta, n}$ $\boxed{+}$ 1 $\boxed{)}$ $\boxed{x^2}$ $\boxed{,}$ $\boxed{\text{X, T, }\Theta, n}$ $\boxed{,}$ 1 $\boxed{,}$ 5 $\boxed{)}$. We will also choose to display the terms of the sequence as fractions by pressing $\boxed{\text{MATH}}$ 1 following the keystrokes shown above. Now press $\boxed{\text{ENTER}}$ to see a list of the first five terms of the sequence. Note that we must use the $\boxed{\triangleright}$ key to see the fourth and fifth terms in the list.

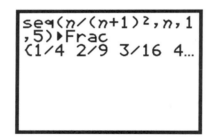
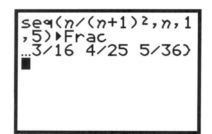

FINDING PARTIAL SUMS

We can use a graphing calculator to find partial sums of a sequence for which the general term is given by a formula.

Section 10.1, Example 5 Use a graphing calculator to find S_1, S_2, S_3, and S_4 for the sequence in which the general term is given by $a_n = (-1)^n/(n+1)$.

We will use the cumSum feature from the LIST OPS menu. This option lists the cumulative, or partial, sums for a sequence defined using the Sequence feature discussed above. First copy cumSum to the home screen by pressing $\boxed{\text{2nd}}$ $\boxed{\text{LIST}}$ $\boxed{\triangleright}$ 6. Next copy the Sequence feature by pressing $\boxed{\text{2nd}}$ $\boxed{\text{LIST}}$ $\boxed{\triangleright}$ 5. Now enter the general term of the sequence, the variable, and the first and last partial sums we wish to calculate, all separated by commas. We will also select the Fraction option from the MATH

MATH menu so that the partial sums will be displayed as fractions. Press $\boxed{(}$ $\boxed{(-)}$ $\boxed{1}$ $\boxed{)}$ $\boxed{\wedge}$ $\boxed{\text{X, T, }\Theta, n}$ $\boxed{\div}$ $\boxed{(}$ $\boxed{\text{X, T, }\Theta, n}$ $\boxed{+}$
$\boxed{1}$ $\boxed{)}$ $\boxed{,}$ $\boxed{\text{X, t, }\Theta, n}$ $\boxed{,}$ $\boxed{1}$ $\boxed{,}$ $\boxed{4}$ $\boxed{)}$ $\boxed{)}$ $\boxed{\text{MATH}}$ $\boxed{1}$ $\boxed{\text{ENTER}}$. Note that we must use the $\boxed{\triangleright}$ key to see S_3 and S_4.

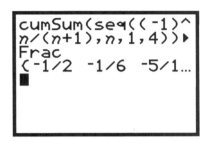   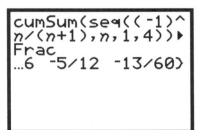

GRAPHS OF SEQUENCES

Section 10.1, Example 8 Graph the sequence for which the general term is given by $a_n = (-1)^n/n$.

The domain of a sequence is a set of integers, so the graph of a sequence is a set of points that are not connected. Thus, we use Dot mode to graph a sequence. Note that the calculator must also be set in Sequence mode.

Press $\boxed{\text{Y} =}$ to go to the sequence-editor screen, and enter $u(n) = (-1)^n/n$ by positioning the cursor beside "$u(n) =$" and pressing $\boxed{(}$ $\boxed{(-)}$ $\boxed{1}$ $\boxed{)}$ $\boxed{\wedge}$ $\boxed{\text{X, T, }\Theta, n}$ $\boxed{\div}$ $\boxed{\text{X, T, }\Theta, n}$. We also let $n\text{Min} = 1$.

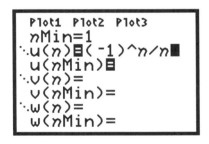

Next we enter the window dimensions. We will graph the sequence from $n = 1$ through $n = 15$, so we let $n\text{Min} = 1$, $n\text{Max} = 15$, $\text{Xmin} = 1$, and $\text{Xmax} = 20$. A table of values of the sequence shows that the terms appear to be between -1 and 1, so we let $\text{Ymin} = -1$ and $\text{Ymax} = 1$ with $\text{Yscl} = 0.1$. We also set both PlotStart and PlotStep to 1. These settings cause the graph to begin with the first term in the sequence and to plot each term of the sequence.

```
WINDOW              WINDOW
 nMin=1              ↑PlotStep=1
 nMax=15              Xmin=0
 PlotStart=1          Xmax=20
 PlotStep=1           Xscl=1
 Xmin=0               Ymin=-1
 Xmax=20              Ymax=1
↓Xscl=1               Yscl=.1
```

Press $\boxed{\text{GRAPH}}$ to see the graph of the sequence.

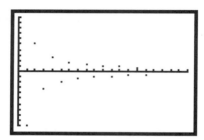

EVALUATING FACTORIALS

Factorials can be evaluated on a graphing calculator.

Section 10.4, Example 3 Simplify: $\dfrac{8!}{5!3!}$.

We use the factorial feature, denoted !, from the MATH PRB (probability) menu. On the home screen press 8 $\boxed{\text{MATH}}$ $\boxed{\triangleleft}$ 4 $\boxed{\div}$ $\boxed{(}$ 5 $\boxed{\text{MATH}}$ $\boxed{\triangleleft}$ 4 3 $\boxed{\text{MATH}}$ $\boxed{\triangleleft}$ 4 $\boxed{)}$ $\boxed{\text{ENTER}}$. Note that we must use parentheses in the denominator so that 8! is divided by both 5! and 3!. We could also access the MATH PRB menu by pressing $\boxed{\text{MATH}}$ $\boxed{\triangleright}$ $\boxed{\triangleright}$ $\boxed{\triangleright}$ rather then $\boxed{\text{MATH}}$ $\boxed{\triangleleft}$, but we used the latter procedure since it requires fewer keystrokes.

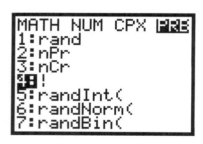
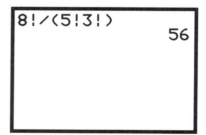

SIMPLIFYING $\left(\begin{array}{c} n \\ r \end{array} \right)$ NOTATION

Section 10.4, Example 4(a) Simplify: $\left(\begin{array}{c} 7 \\ 2 \end{array} \right)$.

The calculator uses the notation ${}_nC_r$ instead of $\left(\begin{array}{c} n \\ r \end{array} \right)$. This option is found in the MATH PRB menu. To simplify $\left(\begin{array}{c} 7 \\ 2 \end{array} \right)$, first press 7, then select option 3 from the MATH PRB menu by pressing $\boxed{\text{MATH}}$ $\boxed{\triangleleft}$ (or $\boxed{\text{MATH}}$ $\boxed{\triangleright}$ $\boxed{\triangleright}$ $\boxed{\triangleright}$) 3, and then press 2 $\boxed{\text{ENTER}}$.

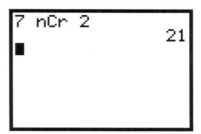

The TI-86
Graphics Calculator

Chapter 1
Basics of Algebra and Graphing

GETTING STARTED

Press ON to turn on the TI-86 graphing calculator. (ON is the key at the bottom left-hand corner of the keypad.) You should see a blinking rectangle, or cursor, on the screen. If you do not see the cursor, try adjusting the display contrast. To do this, first press 2nd. (2nd is the yellow key in the left column of the keypad.) Then press and hold △ to increase the contrast or ▽ to decrease the contrast.

To turn the calculator off, press 2nd OFF. (OFF is the second operation associated with the ON key.) The calculator will turn itself off automatically after about five minutes without any activity.

Press 2nd MODE to display the MODE settings. (MODE is the second operation associated with the MORE key.) Initially you should select the settings on the left side of the display.

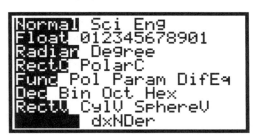

To change a setting on the Mode screen use ▽ or △ to move the cursor to the line of that setting. Then use ▷ or ◁ to move the blinking cursor to the desired setting and press ENTER. Press EXIT, CLEAR, or 2nd QUIT to leave the MODE screen. (QUIT is the second operation associated with the EXIT key.) Pressing EXIT, CLEAR, or 2nd QUIT will take you to the home screen where computations are performed.

It will be helpful to read the Introduction to the Graphing Calculator on pages 9 and 10 of the textbook as well as the Quick Start section and Chapter 1: Operating the TI-86 in your graphing calculator Guidebook before proceeding.

ORDER OF OPERATIONS

The TI-86 follows the rules for order of operations.

Section 1.1, Example 9 Evaluate $2(y - 3)^2 + 7$ for $y = 5$.

Enter the expression on the home screen, substituting 5 for y. Press 2 (5 − 3) x^2 + 7 ENTER. Note that the − key in the right-hand column of the keypad is the subtraction key. The (−) key on the bottom row of the keypad represents "the opposite of" or "the additive inverse of" rather than subtraction. In the expression above we could also have squared $(5 - 3)$ by pressing $\boxed{\wedge}$ 2 rather than $\boxed{x^2}$. The $\boxed{\wedge}$ key indicates exponentiation and the number following it indicates the exponent.

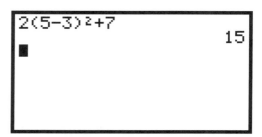

You can recall and edit your entry if necessary. If, for instance, in the expression above you pressed 8 instead of 5, first press $\boxed{\text{2nd}}$ $\boxed{\text{ENTRY}}$ to return to the last entry. (ENTRY is the second operation associated with the $\boxed{\text{ENTER}}$ key.) Then use the $\boxed{\triangleleft}$ key to move the cursor to 8 and press 5 to overwrite it. If you forgot to type the left parenthesis, move the cursor to the 5; then press $\boxed{\text{2nd}}$ $\boxed{\text{INS}}$ $\boxed{(}$ to insert the parenthesis before the 5. (INS, for "insert," is the second operation associated with the $\boxed{\text{DEL}}$ key.) You can continue to insert symbols immediately after the first insertion without pressing $\boxed{\text{2nd}}$ $\boxed{\text{INS}}$ again. If you typed 21 instead of 2, move the cursor to 1 and press $\boxed{\text{DEL}}$. This will delete the 1. If you notice that an entry needs to be edited before you press $\boxed{\text{ENTER}}$ to perform the computation, the editing can be done directly without recalling the entry.

The keystrokes $\boxed{\text{2nd}}$ $\boxed{\text{ENTRY}}$ can be used repeatedly to recall entries preceding the last one. Pressing $\boxed{\text{2nd}}$ $\boxed{\text{ENTRY}}$ twice, for example, will recall the next to last entry. Using these keystrokes a third time recalls the third to last entry and so on. The number of entries that can be recalled depends on the amount of storage they occupy in the calculator's memory.

USING A MENU

A menu is a list of options that appears when a key is pressed. Thus, multiple options, and sometimes multiple menus, may be accessed by pressing one key. For example, the following screen appears when $\boxed{\text{2nd}}$ $\boxed{\text{MATH}}$ is pressed. (MATH is the second operation associated with the $\boxed{\times}$ multiplication key.) We see several submenus at the bottom of the screen. The $\boxed{\text{F1}}$ - $\boxed{\text{F5}}$ keys at the top of the keypad are used to select options from this menu. The arrow to the right of MISC indicates that there are more choices. They can be seen by pressing $\boxed{\text{MORE}}$.

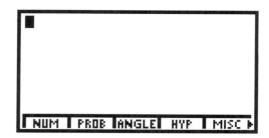

To choose the NUM submenu from the MATH menu press $\boxed{\text{F1}}$. (If you pressed $\boxed{\text{MORE}}$ to see the additional items on the MATH menu as described above, now press $\boxed{\text{MORE}}$ again to see the first five items on the menu. Then press $\boxed{\text{F1}}$ to choose NUM.) When NUM is chosen, the original submenus move up on the screen and the items on the NUM submenu appear at the bottom of the screen.

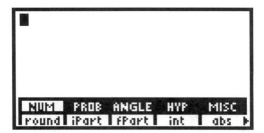

When two rows of options are displayed like this, the top row is accessed by pressing $\boxed{\text{2nd}}$ followed by one of the keys $\boxed{\text{F1}}$ - $\boxed{\text{F5}}$. These keystrokes access the second operations M1 - M5 associated with the $\boxed{\text{F1}}$ - $\boxed{\text{F5}}$ keys. The options on the bottom row are accessed by pressing one of the keys $\boxed{\text{F1}}$ - $\boxed{\text{F5}}$. Absolute value, denoted "abs," is selected from the NUM submenu and copied to the home screen, for instance, by pressing $\boxed{\text{F5}}$.

A menu can be removed from the screen by pressing $\boxed{\text{EXIT}}$. If both a menu and a submenu are displayed, press $\boxed{\text{EXIT}}$ once to remove the submenu and twice to remove both.

The next example involves both order of operations and choosing an option from a menu.

Section 1.2, Example 13 Calculate: $\dfrac{14 - 3| - 16 + 38|}{4| - 2^4 - 3^2|}$.

In order to divide the entire numerator of this fraction by the entire denominator, we must enclose both the numerator and the denominator in parentheses. Recall that the $\boxed{(-)}$ key in the bottom row of the keypad must be used to enter a negative number on the calculator whereas the $\boxed{-}$ key is used to enter subtraction. Also remember that absolute value notation is found on the MATH NUM menu.

To enter the expression above, press $\boxed{(}$ 1 4 $\boxed{-}$ 3 $\boxed{\text{2nd}}$ $\boxed{\text{MATH}}$ $\boxed{\text{F1}}$ $\boxed{\text{F5}}$ $\boxed{(}$ $\boxed{(-)}$ 1 6 $\boxed{+}$ 3 8 $\boxed{)}$ $\boxed{)}$ $\boxed{\div}$ $\boxed{(}$ $\boxed{(}$ 4 $\boxed{\text{F5}}$ $\boxed{(}$ $\boxed{(-)}$ 2 $\boxed{\wedge}$ 4 $\boxed{-}$ 3 $\boxed{x^2}$ $\boxed{)}$ $\boxed{)}$ $\boxed{)}$ $\boxed{\text{ENTER}}$.

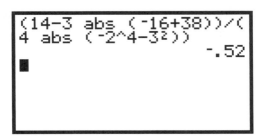

Note that the entire numerator and the entire denominator must be enclosed in parentheses. The absolute value expressions in both the numerator and the denominator must be enclosed in parentheses as well.

The result of the calculation above can be converted from decimal notation to fractional notation by pressing $\boxed{\text{2nd}}$ $\boxed{\text{MATH}}$ $\boxed{\text{F5}}$ $\boxed{\text{MORE}}$ $\boxed{\text{F1}}$ $\boxed{\text{ENTER}}$. These keystrokes tell the calculator to use the previous answer, and then they access the MATH MISC menu, copy the item "▷ Frac" to the home screen, and display the conversion. The keystroke $\boxed{\text{F5}}$ selects the MISC submenu from the MATH menu, and $\boxed{\text{F1}}$ selects ▷ Frac from the MATH MISC submenu. Note that this must be done immediately after the calculation is performed in order to have the result of the calculation available for the conversion.

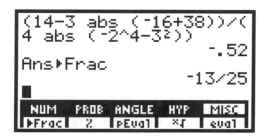

If only a fractional answer is desired, the keystrokes 2nd MATH F5 MORE F1 can be inserted before the final ENTER in the computation and a fractional answer will be displayed immediately.

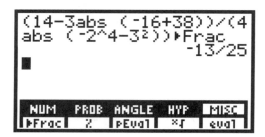

Absolute value notation can also be found as the first item in the CATALOG and copied to the home screen. To do this press 2nd CATLG-VARS F1 ENTER . (CATALOG is the second operation associated with the CUSTOM key. A is the blue alphabetic operation associated with the LOG key.) Pressing A takes us to the first item in the Catalog that begins with A. A triangular selection cursor will be positioned beside the item "abs." Press ENTER to copy this item to the home screen. If the cursor is positioned beside "abs" after F1 is pressed above, it is not necessary to press A .

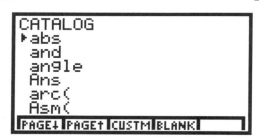

THE CUSTOM MENU

The TI-86 allows you to create a custom menu containing up to 15 items selected from the Catalog. To display the custom menu, press CUSTOM .

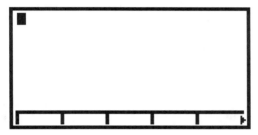

Press MORE once to see the second menu group and press MORE once again to see the third group.

To clear an item from the custom menu, press 2nd CATLG-VARS F1 F4 to select BLANK from the Catalog menu. Then press one of the F1 - F5 keys corresponding to the location of the item to be cleared. To clear an item in the middle position of the first custom menu group, for instance, press F3 . To clear an item in the second or third menu group, press MORE once or twice before pressing one of the F1 - F5 keys. A new item added to a custom menu will replace the item currently in that location, so it is not necessary to clear an item before one is added in its place.

We will put "abs" and "▷ Frac" in a custom menu to illustrate the procedure. To place "abs" in position F1 of the first menu group, first select Custom from the catalog menu be pressing 2nd CATLG-VARS F1 F3 . Now move the triangular selection cursor in the Catalog to the first item that begins with A by pressing A . That item is "abs." Copy it to position F1 in the custom menu by pressing F1 .

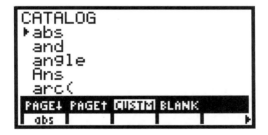

To enter "▷ Frac" in position F2, first use ▽ to position the triangular cursor beside "▷ Frac" in the Catalog. This item follows the items beginning with Z as well as a large number of symbolic items. Then press F2 to copy the item to position F2.

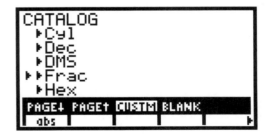 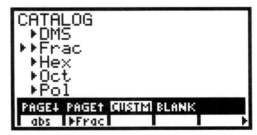

SCIENTIFIC NOTATION

To enter a number in scientific notation, first type the decimal portion of the number; then press $\boxed{\text{EE}}$; finally type the exponent, which can be at most two digits. For example, to enter 1.789×10^{-11} in scientific notation, press 1 $\boxed{.}$ $7\ 8\ 9$ $\boxed{\text{EE}}$ $\boxed{(-)}$ $1\ 1$ $\boxed{\text{ENTER}}$. To enter 6.084×10^{23} in scientific notation, press 6 $\boxed{.}$ $0\ 8\ 4$ $\boxed{\text{EE}}$ $2\ 3$ $\boxed{\text{ENTER}}$. The decimal portion of each number appears before a small E while the exponent follows the E.

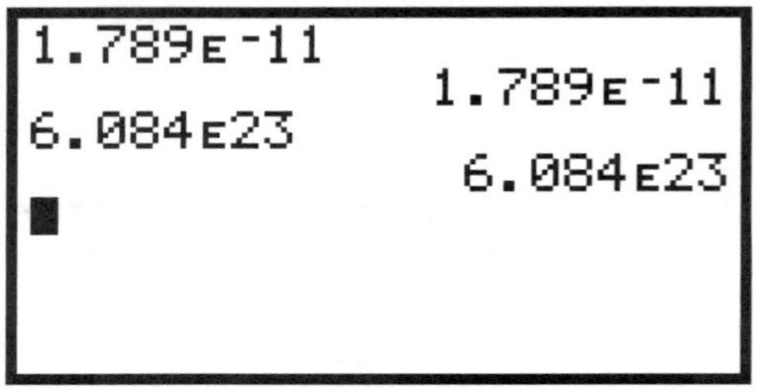

```
1.789E-11
6.084E23                 1.789E-11
■                        6.084E23
```

The calculator can be used to perform computations in scientific notation.

Section 1.4, Example 14 Use a graphing calculator to check the computation $(7.2 \times 10^5)(4.3 \times 10^9) = 3.096 \times 10^{15}$.

We enter the computation in scientific notation. Press 7 $\boxed{.}$ 2 $\boxed{\text{EE}}$ 5 $\boxed{\times}$ 4 $\boxed{.}$ 3 $\boxed{\text{EE}}$ 9 $\boxed{\text{ENTER}}$. We have 3.096×10^{15}, which checks.

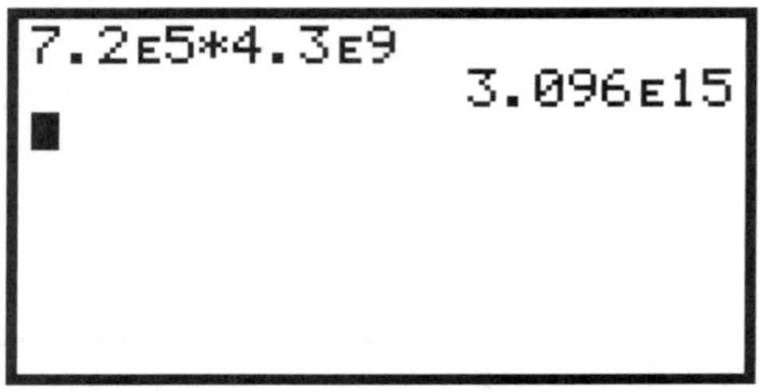

```
7.2E5*4.3E9
■                     3.096E15
```

SETTING THE VIEWING WINDOW

The viewing window is the portion of the coordinate plane that appears on the graphing calculator's screen. It is defined by the minimum and maximum values of x and y: xMin, xMax, yMin, and yMax. The notation [xMin, xMax, yMin, yMax] is used in the text to represent these window settings or dimensions. For example, $[-12, 12, -8, 8]$ denotes a window that displays the portion of the x-axis from -12 to 12 and the portion of the y-axis from -8 to 8. In addition, the distance between tick marks on the axes is defined by the settings xScl and yScl. In this manual xScl and yScl will be assumed to be 1 unless noted otherwise. The setting xRes sets the pixel resolution. We usually select Xres = 1. The window corresponding to the settings $[-20, 30, -12, 20]$, xScl = 5, yScl = 2, xRes = 1, is shown below.

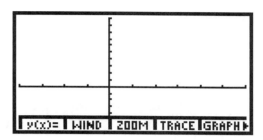

Press $\boxed{\text{GRAPH}}$ $\boxed{\text{F2}}$ key to display the current window settings on your calculator in the WINDOW screen. The standard settings are shown below.

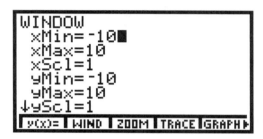 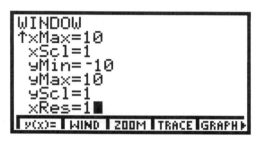

To change a setting, position the cursor beside the setting you wish to change and enter the new value. For example, to change from the standard settings to $[-20, 30, -12, 20]$, xScl $= 5$, yScl $= 2$, on the WINDOW screen press $\boxed{(-)}$ 2 0 $\boxed{\text{ENTER}}$ 3 0 $\boxed{\text{ENTER}}$ 5 $\boxed{\text{ENTER}}$ $\boxed{(-)}$ 1 2 $\boxed{\text{ENTER}}$ 2 0 $\boxed{\text{ENTER}}$ 2 $\boxed{\text{ENTER}}$. The $\boxed{\triangledown}$ key may be used instead of $\boxed{\text{ENTER}}$ after typing each window setting. To see the window, press the $\boxed{\text{GRAPH}}$ key on the top row of the keypad. This is the window shown above.

QUICK TIP: To return quickly to the standard window setting $[-10, 10, -10, 10]$, xScl $= 1$, yScl $= 1$, press $\boxed{\text{GRAPH}}$ $\boxed{\text{F3}}$ $\boxed{\text{F4}}$.

GRAPHING EQUATIONS

After entering an equation and setting a viewing window, you can view the graph of an equation.

Section 1.5, Example 5 Graph $y = 2x$ using a graphing calculator.

Equations are entered on the equation-editor screen. Press $\boxed{\text{GRAPH}}$ $\boxed{\text{F1}}$ to access this screen. If there is currently an expression displayed for $y1$, clear it by positioning the cursor beside "$y1 =$" and pressing $\boxed{\text{CLEAR}}$. Do the same for expressions that appear on all other lines by using $\boxed{\triangledown}$ to move to a line and then pressing $\boxed{\text{CLEAR}}$. Note the any Stat Plots that had previously been turned on should be turned off. The names of the plots that are turned on are highlighted on the equation-editor screen. To turn off a plot, position the cursor over its name and press $\boxed{\text{ENTER}}$. Plots can also be turned off from the STAT menu as described above.

To enter the equation, first use $\boxed{\triangle}$ or $\boxed{\triangledown}$ to move the cursor beside "$y1 =$." Now press 2 $\boxed{\text{x-VAR}}$ or 2 $\boxed{\text{F1}}$ to enter the right-hand side of the equation in the equation-editor screen. Note that the variable x can be entered either by pressing the $\boxed{\text{x-VAR}}$ key or by pressing $\boxed{\text{F1}}$ to select x from the $y(x) =$ submenu on the equation-editor screen.

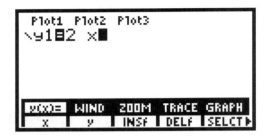

The standard $[-10, 10, -10, 10]$ window is a good choice for this graph. Enter these dimensions in the WINDOW screen and then press $\boxed{\text{F5}}$ to see the graph or, from the equation-editor screen, simply press $\boxed{\text{2nd}}$ $\boxed{\text{F3}}$ $\boxed{\text{F4}}$ to select the standard window and see the graph. To remove the menu from the bottom of the screen, press $\boxed{\text{CLEAR}}$. The menu will reappear when $\boxed{\text{GRAPH}}$ is pressed.

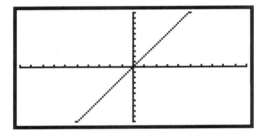

THE TABLE FEATURE

For an equation entered in the equation-editor screen, a table of x-and y-values can be displayed.

Section 1.5, Example 7 Create a table of ordered pairs that are solutions of the equation $y = -\dfrac{1}{2}x$. Use integer values of x beginning at -3.

First press $\boxed{\text{GRAPH}}$ $\boxed{\text{F1}}$ to access the equation-editor screen. Then clear any equations that are present. (See Example 5 above for the procedure to follow.) Next enter the equation by positioning the cursor beside "$y1 =$" and pressing $\boxed{(-)}$ $\boxed{(}$ 1 $\boxed{\div}$ 2 $\boxed{)}$ $\boxed{\text{F1}}$. Although the parentheses are not necessary on the TI-86, the equation is more easily read when they are used.

Once the equation in entered, press the $\boxed{\text{TABLE}}$ key in the second column of the keypad followed by $\boxed{\text{F2}}$ to access the TABLE SETUP screen. You can choose to supply the x-values yourself or you can set the calculator to supply them.

If "Indpnt" is set to "Auto," the calculator will supply values for x, beginning with the value specified as TblStart and continuing by adding the value of ΔTbl to the preceding value for x. For example, for the equation $y = -\dfrac{1}{2}x$ entered above, we will set the table to Auto mode and display a table of values that starts with $x = -3$ and adds 1 to the preceding x-value. Press -3 $\boxed{\triangledown}$ 1 to select a minimum x-value of -3 and an increment of 1. The "Indpnt" setting should be "Auto." If it is not, use the $\boxed{\triangledown}$ key to position the blinking cursor over "Auto" and then press $\boxed{\text{ENTER}}$. To display the table press $\boxed{\text{F1}}$. The $\boxed{\triangle}$ and $\boxed{\triangledown}$ keys can be used to scroll through the table.

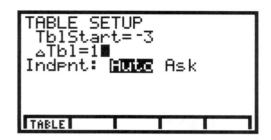

GRAPHS AS MODELS

A graphing calculator can plot data points and draw a line graph using those points.

Section 1.6, Example 7 *Weekly Newspapers.* The following table show the number of weekly newspapers in the United States for various years from 1960 to 2000. Use the data to draw a line graph.

Year	Number of Weekday Newspapers
1960	8174
1970	7612
1980	7954
1990	7606
2000	7689

We will enter the coordinates of the ordered pairs on the STAT list editor screen. To clear any existing lists first press $\boxed{\text{2nd}}$ $\boxed{\text{STAT}}$ $\boxed{\text{F2}}$ (for EDIT). (STAT is the second operation associated with the $\boxed{+}$ key.) Then use the arrow keys to move up to highlight "xStat" and press $\boxed{\text{CLEAR}}$ $\boxed{\text{ENTER}}$. Do the same for yStat.

Once the lists are cleared, we can enter the coordinates of the points. We will enter the first coordinates (x-coordinates) in xStat and the second coordinates (y-coordinates) in yStat. Position the cursor at the top of column xStat, below the xStat heading. To enter 1960 press 1 9 6 0 $\boxed{\text{ENTER}}$. Continue typing the x-values 1970, 1980, 1990, and 2000, each followed by $\boxed{\text{ENTER}}$. The entries can be followed by $\boxed{\triangledown}$ rather than $\boxed{\text{ENTER}}$ if desired. Press $\boxed{\triangleright}$ to move to the top of column yStat. Type the y-values 8174, 7612, 7954, 7606, and 7689 in succession, each followed by $\boxed{\text{ENTER}}$ or $\boxed{\triangledown}$. Note that the coordinates of each point must be in the same position in both lists.

To plot the points, we turn on the STAT PLOT feature. To access the STAT PLOT screen, press $\boxed{\text{2nd}}$ $\boxed{\text{STAT}}$ $\boxed{\text{F3}}$.

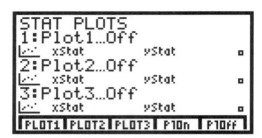

Choose Plot 1 by pressing $\boxed{\text{F1}}$. Now position the cursor over On and press $\boxed{\text{ENTER}}$ to turn on Plot 1. The entries Type, Xlist, and Ylist, and Mark should be as shown below. To select Type, use the $\boxed{\bigtriangledown}$ key to position the cursor beside Type = and then press one the keys $\boxed{\text{F1}}$ - $\boxed{\text{F5}}$. Here we pressed $\boxed{\text{F2}}$ to select xyLINE for a line graph. Use the $\boxed{\bigtriangledown}$ key again to position the cursor beside Xlist Name = and press $\boxed{\text{F1}}$ to select xStat. Select yStat for Ylist similarly. The last item, Mark, allows us to choose a box, a cross, or a dot for each point. Here we have selected a box by positioning the cursor beside Mark = and pressing $\boxed{\text{F1}}$.

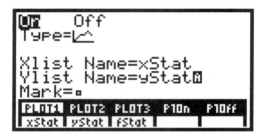

Note that there should be no equations entered on the "$y =$" screen. Press $\boxed{\text{GRAPH}}$ $\boxed{\text{F1}}$ to go to this screen. If there are entries present clear them now. (See page 65 of this manual for instructions on clearing equations.) If this is not done, the equations that are currently entered will be graphed along with the data points that are entered.

Now enter a viewing window that will display all the data points. The years range from 1960 to 2000 and the numbers of newspapers range from 7606 to 8174, so one good choice is $[1950, 2010, 7500, 8500]$, xScl $=10$, yScl $= 100$. From the WINDOW screen press $\boxed{\text{F5}}$ to see the line graph of the data. The ZData option will automatically select a window that shows all the data points. Activate this option by pressing $\boxed{\text{GRAPH}}$ $\boxed{\text{F3}}$ $\boxed{\text{MORE}}$ $\boxed{\text{F5}}$.

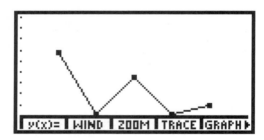

THE TRACE FEATURE

The graphing calculator's Trace feature displays the coordinates of the point indicated by the cursor.

Section 1.6, Example 8 *Model Rockets.* Suppose that a model rocket is launched upward with an initial velocity of 96 ft/sec. Its height in feet, h, after t seconds is given by

$$h = -16t^2 + 96t.$$

(a) For how long will the rocket climb?

(b) How high will the rocket go?

(c) After how long will the rocket reach the ground?

First we press $\boxed{\text{GRAPH}}$ $\boxed{\text{F1}}$ to go to the equation-editor screen. Enter $Y_1 = -16x^2 + 96x$ and graph the equation in the viewing window $[0, 10, 0, 200]$, yScl $= 10$. Note that the Stat Plots should be turned off. (See page 72 of this manual for the procedure.)

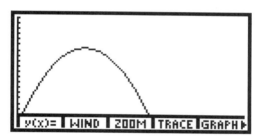

(a) The rocket climbs until the graph reaches the greatest y-value. The x-value associated with this y-value indicates how long the rocket climbs. To find this value, press $\boxed{\text{F4}}$. The trace cursor appears on the graph. Use the right and left arrow keys to move the cursor to the highest point on the graph. The greatest y-value occurs when x is about 3, so we can say that the rocket climbs for about 3 seconds.

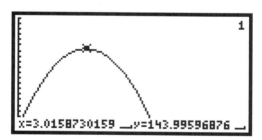

(b) To approximate how high the rocket will go, we read the greatest y-value in the Trace window above. Thus, we would say that the rocket will go to a height of about 144 feet.

(c) The rocket is on the ground when $y = 0$. The x-value associated with this y-value indicates how long it will take the rocket to reach the ground. We use Trace to find this x-value. Press $\boxed{\text{GRAPH}}$ $\boxed{\text{F4}}$ and use the right arrow key to move the cursor to the point on the right side of the graph where y is approximately 0. We see that this y-value occurs when x is about 6, so we say that is will take about 6 seconds for the rocket to reach the ground.

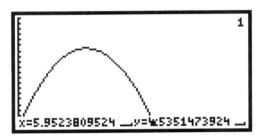

Chapter 2
Functions, Linear Equations, and Models

EVALUATING A FUNCTION

Function values can be found in several different ways on the TI-86.

Section 2.1, Example 6 For $f(a) = 2a^2 - 3a + 1$, find $f(3)$ and $f(-5.1)$.

One method for finding function values involves using function notation directly. To do this, first press $\boxed{\text{GRAPH}}$ $\boxed{\text{F1}}$ and enter the function on the equation-editor screen. Mentally replace a with x and $f(a)$ with $y1$. Then enter $y1 = 2x^2 - 3x + 1$. Now, to find $f(3)$, or $y1(3)$, directly first press $\boxed{\text{2nd}}$ $\boxed{\text{QUIT}}$ to go to the home screen. Then press $\boxed{\text{2nd}}$ $\boxed{\text{CATLG-VARS}}$ $\boxed{\text{MORE}}$ $\boxed{\text{F4}}$. If the triangular selection cursor is not positioned beside $y1$, use the $\boxed{\triangle}$ key to move it there. Now press $\boxed{\text{ENTER}}$ to paste $y1$ to the home screen and then press $\boxed{(}$ 3 $\boxed{)}$ $\boxed{\text{ENTER}}$. We see that $y1(3) = 10$, or $f(3) = 10$.

To find $f(-5.1)$, or $y1(-5.1)$, we can repeat the previous procedure using -5.1 in place of 3, or we can edit the previous entry. To edit, copy the entry $y1(3)$ to the home screen by pressing $\boxed{\text{2nd}}$ $\boxed{\text{ENTRY}}$. Now replace 3 with -5.1 by first pressing $\boxed{\triangleleft}$ $\boxed{\triangleleft}$ to position the cursor over the 3. Then press $\boxed{(-)}$ to overwrite the 3 with the negative symbol. To insert 5.1 after this symbol press $\boxed{\text{2nd}}$ $\boxed{\text{INS}}$ 5 $\boxed{.}$ 1. Finally press $\boxed{\text{ENTER}}$ to find that $y1(-5.1) = 68.32$, or $f(-5.1) = 68.32$.

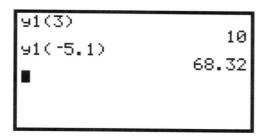

Another way to calculate a function value after the function has been entered on the equation-editor screen involves storing the input value in the calculator's memory. To find $f(3)$ for the function entered as $y1$ in this example, for instance, we can store 3 as the variable X by pressing 3 $\boxed{\text{STO} \triangleright}$ $\boxed{\text{x-VAR}}$ $\boxed{\text{ENTER}}$. Then select $y1$ by first pressing $\boxed{\text{2nd}}$ $\boxed{\text{CATLG-VARS}}$ $\boxed{\text{MORE}}$ $\boxed{\text{F4}}$. Position the triangular cursor beside $y1$ and then press $\boxed{\text{ENTER}}$ $\boxed{\text{ENTER}}$ to find the value of $y1$ when $x = 3$.

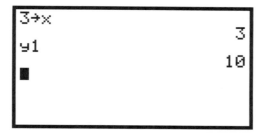

This computation can also be performed in a single step by first pressing 3 $\boxed{\text{STO} \rhd}$ $\boxed{x\text{-VAR}}$ $\boxed{\text{2nd}}$ $\boxed{:}$ $\boxed{\text{2nd}}$ $\boxed{\text{CATLG-VARS}}$ $\boxed{\text{MORE}}$ $\boxed{\text{F4}}$. Then position the triangular cursor beside $y1$ and press $\boxed{\text{ENTER}}$ $\boxed{\text{ENTER}}$ (The symbol : is the second operation associated with the $\boxed{.}$ key.)

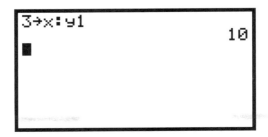

We can also find function values from the graph of the function.

Section 2.1, Example 7 Find $g(2)$ for $g(x) = 2x - 5$.

First press $\boxed{\text{GRAPH}}$ $\boxed{\text{F1}}$ to go to the equation editor screen and then clear any entries that are present. Also be sure that the Stat Plots are turned off. (See page 65 of this manual for instructions for clearing equations and turning off Stat Plots.) Now enter $y1 = 2x - 5$ and press $\boxed{\text{2nd}}$ $\boxed{\text{F3}}$ $\boxed{\text{F4}}$ to graph this function in the standard viewing window. We will use the EVAL feature from the GRAPH menu to find the value of $y1$ when $x = 2$. This is $g(2)$. From the Graph window press $\boxed{\text{MORE}}$ $\boxed{\text{MORE}}$ $\boxed{\text{F1}}$ to select EVAL. (If you pressed $\boxed{\text{CLEAR}}$ to remove the menu from the Graph screen, press $\boxed{\text{GRAPH}}$ first.) Now you must supply the value of x as indicated by the blinking cursor at the bottom of the screen beside x =. Press 2 $\boxed{\text{ENTER}}$. We now see X = 2, Y = −1 at the bottom of the screen, so $g(2) = -1$.

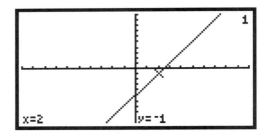

When using the EVAL feature, note that the x-value entered must be in the viewing window. That is, x must be a number between xMin and xMax.

SOLVING EQUATIONS GRAPHICALLY

We can use the Intersect feature from the GRAPH menu to solve equations.

Section 2.2, Example 3 Solve using a graphing calculator: $-\dfrac{3}{4}x + 6 = 2x - 1$.

On the equation editor screen, clear any existing entries and then enter $y1 = -(3/4)x + 6$ and $y2 = 2x - 1$. (Press $\boxed{\triangledown}$ or $\boxed{\text{ENTER}}$ after entering $y1$ to position the cursor beside $y2 =$.) Although the parentheses in $y1$ are not necessary, they make the equation easier to read on the equation-editor screen. Press $\boxed{\text{2nd}}$ $\boxed{\text{M3}}$ $\boxed{\text{F4}}$ to graph these equations in the standard viewing window. The solution of the equation $-\frac{3}{4}x + 6 = 2x - 1$ is the first coordinate of the point of intersection of these graphs. To use the Intersect feature to find this point, from the Graph screen first press $\boxed{\text{MORE}}$ $\boxed{\text{F1}}$ $\boxed{\text{MORE}}$ $\boxed{\text{F3}}$ to select ISECT from the GRAPH MATH menu. The query "First curve?" appears at the bottom of the screen. The blinking cursor is positioned on the graph of $y1$. This is indicated by the number 1 in the upper right-hand corner of the screen. Press $\boxed{\text{ENTER}}$ to indicate that this is the first curve involved in the intersection. Next the query "Second curve?" appears at the bottom of the screen. The blinking cursor is now positioned on the graph of $y2$, indicated by the number 2 appearing in the top right-hand corner of the screen. Press $\boxed{\text{ENTER}}$ to indicate that this is the second curve. We identify the curves since we could have as many as ten graphs on the screen at once. After we identify the second curve, the query "Guess?" appears at the bottom of the screen. Use the right and left arrow keys to move the blinking cursor close to the point of intersection of the graphs or type a number that approximates the first coordinate of the point of intersection. This provides the calculator with a guess as to the coordinates of this point. We do this since some pairs of curves can have more than one point of intersection. When the cursor is positioned or the approximation is typed, press $\boxed{\text{ENTER}}$ a third time. Now the coordinates of the point of intersection appear at the bottom of the screen.

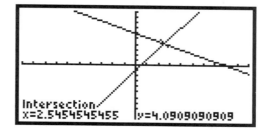

We see that $x = 2.5454545455$, so the solution of the equation is 2.5454545455.

We can check the solution by evaluating both sides of the equation $-\frac{3}{4}x + 6 = 2x - 1$ for this value of x. The first coordinate of the point of intersection has automatically been stored as x in the calculator, so we evaluate $y1$ and $y2$ for this value of x. First press $\boxed{\text{2nd}}$ $\boxed{\text{QUIT}}$ to go to the home screen. Then to evaluate $y1$ press $\boxed{\text{2nd}}$ $\boxed{\text{CATLG-VARS}}$ $\boxed{\text{MORE}}$ $\boxed{\text{F4}}$, position the triangular selection cursor beside $y1$, and press $\boxed{\text{ENTER}}$ $\boxed{\text{ENTER}}$. Repeat this procedure for $y2$, positioning the triangular cursor beside $y2$ this time. We see that $y1$ and $y2$ have the same value when x = 2.5454545455, so the solution checks.

```
y1
              4.09090909091
y2
              4.09090909091
■
```

Note that although the procedure above verifies that 2.5454545455 is the solution, it is actually an approximation of the solution. To find the exact solution we can solve the equation algebraically.

SOLVING FOR Y

The TI-86 graphs only functions, so an equation must be solved for the dependent variable before it can be entered into the calculator.

Section 2.3, Example 8 Graph $3x - 4y = 2y + 7$.

We must first use our formula-solving skills to solve this equation for y. We get $y = \dfrac{-3x + 7}{-6}$. Since $y = \dfrac{-3x + 7}{-6}$ is equivalent to $3x - 4y = 2y + 7$, the graphs of these equations will be the same. Thus, we can enter the equation $y1 = (-3x + 7)/(-6)$ on the equation-editor screen. Note that, although the parentheses in the denominator are not necessary on the TI-86, they make the equation easier to read on the equation-editor screen. We graph the equation in the standard viewing window.

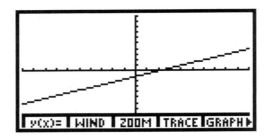

SQUARING THE VIEWING WINDOW

Section 2.5, Example 8 Determine whether the lines given by the equations $3x - y = 7$ and $x + 3y = 1$ are perpendicular, and check by graphing.

In the text each equation is solved for y in order to determine the slopes of the lines. We have $y = 3x - 7$ and $y = -\dfrac{1}{3}x + \dfrac{1}{3}$. Since $3\left(-\dfrac{1}{3}\right) = -1$, we know that the lines are perpendicular. To check this, we graph $y1 = 3x - 7$ and $y2 = -\dfrac{1}{3}x + \dfrac{1}{3}$. The graphs are shown below in the standard viewing window.

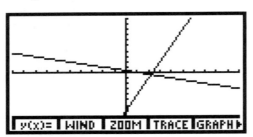

Note that the graphs do not appear to be perpendicular. This is due to the fact that, in the standard window, the distance between tick marks on the y-axis is about 3/5 the distance between tick marks on the x-axis. It is often desirable to choose window dimensions for which these distances are the same, creating a "square" window. On the TI-86, any window in which the ratio of the length of the y-axis to the length of the x-axis is 3/5 will produce this effect.

This can be accomplished by selecting dimensions for which yMax $-$ yMin $= \dfrac{3}{5}$(xMax $-$ xMin). For example, the windows $[-20, 20, -12, 12]$ and $[-10, 10, -6, 6]$ are square. When we change the dimensions to $[-10, 10, -6, 6]$ and press $\boxed{\text{GRAPH}}$ $\boxed{\text{F5}}$, the graphs now appear to be perpendicular as shown on the right below.

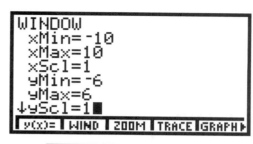 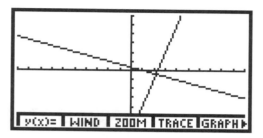

We could also press GRAPH ZOOM MORE F2 and the calculator will select a square window.

LINEAR REGRESSION

We can use the Linear Regression feature in the STAT CALC menu to fit a linear equation to a set of data.

Section 2.6, Example 5 The amount of paper recovered in the United States for various years is shown in the following table.

Years	Amount of Paper Recovered (in millions of tons)
1988	26.2
1990	29.1
1992	34.0
1994	39.7
1996	43.1
1998	45.1
2000	49.4

(a) Fit a linear function to the data.

(b) Graph the function and use it to estimate the amount of paper that will be recovered in 2003.

(a) Press 2nd STAT F2 to display the STAT lists. Clear any data previously entered in the lists and then enter data with the number of years since 1988 in xStat and the number of millions of tons of paper recovered in yStat. (See page 67 of this manual for the procedure to follow to do this.)

Now press GRAPH F1 to go to the equation-editor screen and clear any equations that are currently entered. (See page 65 of this manual.) If you wish, instead of clearing an equation, you can deselect it. To do this, position the cursor beside the = sign and press F5. Note that the = sign is no longer highlighted, indicating that the equation has been deselected. The graph of an equation that has been deselected will not appear when the Graph screen is displayed. A deselected equation can be selected again by positioning the cursor beside the = sign and pressing F5. Note that the = sign is once again highlighted.

Now use the graphing calculator's linear regression feature to fit a linear equation to the data. Go to the home screen and press $\boxed{\text{2nd}}$ $\boxed{\text{STAT}}$ $\boxed{\text{F1}}$ $\boxed{\text{F3}}$ to select linear regression, LinR, from the STAT CALC menu. Next enter the names of the lists that contain the variables x and y. Press $\boxed{\text{2nd}}$ $\boxed{\text{LIST}}$ $\boxed{\text{F3}}$ $\boxed{\text{F2}}$ $\boxed{,}$ $\boxed{\text{F3}}$. Finally, press $\boxed{\text{ENTER}}$ to see the coefficients of the regression equation $y = a + bx$. W see that the regression equation is $y = 1.97678571x + 26.225$.

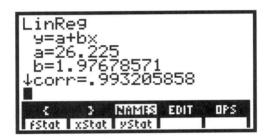

Note that we also see the coefficient of correlation, denoted "corr." This number indicates how well the regression line fits the data. Press $\boxed{\text{EXIT}}$ to remove the STAT CALC menu and display n, the number of data points. We have pressed $\boxed{\text{EXIT}}$ twice to produce the screen below.

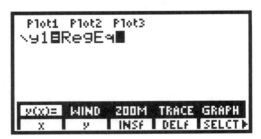

Immediately after the regression equation is found it can be copied to the equation-editor screen as $y1$. Note that any previous entry in $y1$ must have been cleared rather than deselected. Press $\boxed{\text{GRAPH}}$ $\boxed{\text{F1}}$ and position the cursor beside $y1$. Then press $\boxed{\text{2nd}}$ $\boxed{\text{CATLG-VARS}}$ $\boxed{\text{MORE}}$ $\boxed{\text{MORE}}$ $\boxed{\text{F4}}$, use the $\boxed{\triangledown}$ key to position the cursor beside RegEq, and press $\boxed{\text{ENTER}}$. These keystrokes select the VARIABLES:STAT submenu from the CATLG-VARS menu, then select RegEq (Regression Equation) from this submenu, and paste it to the equation-editor screen.

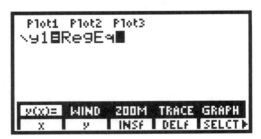

Before the regression equation is found, it is possible to select a y-variable to which it will be stored on the equation-editor screen. After the data have been stored in the lists and the equation previously entered as $y1$ has been cleared, press $\boxed{\text{2nd}}$ $\boxed{\text{STAT}}$ $\boxed{\text{F1}}$ $\boxed{\text{F3}}$ $\boxed{\text{2nd}}$ $\boxed{\text{LIST}}$ $\boxed{\text{F3}}$ $\boxed{\text{F2}}$ $\boxed{,}$ $\boxed{\text{F3}}$ $\boxed{,}$ $\boxed{\text{2nd}}$ $\boxed{\text{alpha}}$ $\boxed{\text{Y}}$ $\boxed{1}$ $\boxed{\text{ENTER}}$. (Y is the blue alphabetic operation associated with the

0 numeric key.) The coefficients of the regression equation will be displayed on the home screen, and the regression equation will also be stored as $y1$ on the equation-editor screen.

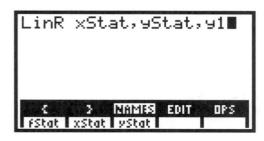 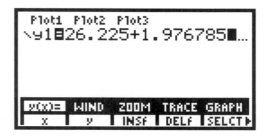

(b) Now we will graph the regression equation. In order to see the data points along with the graph of the equation we will turn on and define a Stat Plot. To do this, press $\boxed{\text{2nd}}$ $\boxed{\text{STAT}}$ $\boxed{\text{F3}}$ to go to the STAT PLOT screen. Press $\boxed{\text{F1}}$ to select Plot 1 and then press $\boxed{\text{ENTER}}$ to turn on Plot 1. Next select the scatter diagram for Type, xStat for Xlist Name, yStat for Ylist Name, and the box for the Mark as shown below. (See pages 67 and 68 of this manual for instructions.)

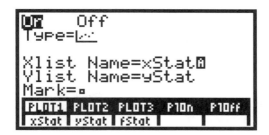

To select the dimensions of the viewing window notice that the years in the table range from 0 to 12 and the number of millions of tons of paper ranges from 26.2 to 49.4. We want to select dimensions that will include all of these values. One good choice is [0, 15, 0, 60], Yscl =10. Press $\boxed{\text{GRAPH}}$ $\boxed{\text{F2}}$ and enter these dimensions in the WINDOW screen.

Since the regression equation has been copied to the equation-editor screen, we can now press $\boxed{\text{GRAPH}}$ $\boxed{\text{F5}}$ to graph the regression line on the same axes as the data. Recall that, instead of entering window dimensions directly, from the Plot 1 screen we can press $\boxed{\text{GRAPH}}$ $\boxed{\text{F3}}$ $\boxed{\text{MORE}}$ $\boxed{\text{F5}}$ to activate the ZData operation which automatically selects a viewing window that contains all of the data points and also displays the graph.

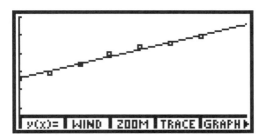

To estimate the amount of paper that will be recovered in 2003, evaluate the regression equation for $x = 15$. (2003 is 15 years after 1988.) The FCST (Forecast) feature from the STAT menu lends itself well to evaluating regression functions. Press $\boxed{\text{2nd}}$

STAT MORE F1 . The blinking cursor appears beside $x =$. Enter 15 for x by pressing 1 5 ENTER . Now the cursor is positioned beside $y =$. Press F5 to see the value of y when $x = 15$. Instead of using the FCST feature, we could have used any of the methods for evaluating a function presented earlier in this chapter. (See pages 71 and 72.) We see that when $x = 15, y \approx 55.9$, so we estimate that about 55.9 million tons of paper will be recovered in 2003.

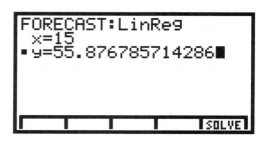

Chapter 3
Systems of Equations and Problem Solving

SOLVING SYSTEMS OF EQUATIONS GRAPHICALLY

We can use the Intersect feature from the GRAPH MATH menu on the TI-86 to solve a system of two equations in two variables.

Section 3.1, Example 4(a) Solve graphically:

$$y - x = 1,$$

$$y + x = 3.$$

We graph the equations in the same viewing window and then find the coordinates of the point of intersection. Remember that equations must be entered in "$y =$" form on the equation-editor screen, so we solve both equations for y. We have $y = x + 1$ and $y = -x + 3$. Enter these equations, graph them in the standard viewing window, and find their point of intersection as described on pages 72 and 73 of this manual. We see that the solution of the system of equations is $(1, 2)$.

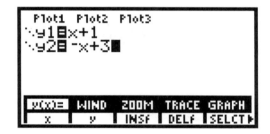 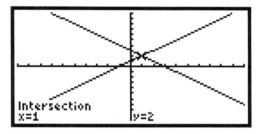

MODELS

Sometimes we model two situations with linear functions and then want to find the point of intersection of their graphs.

Section 3.1, Example 6 (d), (e) The numbers of U. S. travelers to Canada and to Europe are listed in the following table.

Year	U. S. Travelers to Canada (in millions)	U. S. Travelers to Europe (in millions)
1992	11.8	7.1
1994	12.5	8.2
1996	12.9	8.7
1998	14.9	11.1
2000	15.1	13.4

(d) Use linear regression to find two linear equations that can be used to estimate the number of U. S. travelers to Canada and Europe, in millions, x years after 1990.

(e) Use the equations found in part (d) to estimate the year in which the number of U. S. travelers to Europe will be the same as the number of U. S. travelers to Canada.

(d) To find the function $w(t)$, we enter the data for the years and waste generated in STAT lists as described on page 67 of this manual. We will express the years as the number of years after 1990 (in other words, 1990 is year 0) and enter them in xStat. Then enter the number of travelers to Canada, in millions, in yStat.

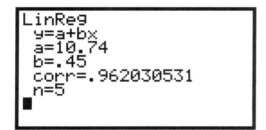

Now use linear regression to fit a linear function to the data. The function should also be copied to the equation editor screen. We will copy it as $y1$. See pages 76 and 77 of this manual for the procedure to follow. We get $y1 = 10.74 + 0.45x$, or $y1 = 0.45x + 10.74$.

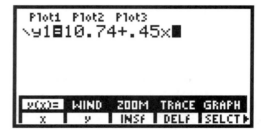

Next we fit a linear function to the data for the number of travelers to Europe, in millions, and save it as $y2$ on the equation-editor screen. We keep the number of years after 1990 in xStat and enter the number of travelers to Europe, in millions, in yStat.

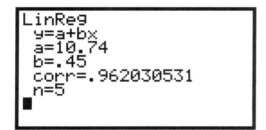

After entering the data, press EXIT to go to the home screen. Then press 2nd STAT F1 F3 2nd LIST F3 F2 , F3 , 2nd ALPHA Y 2 ENTER. We get $y2 = 5.05 + 0.775x$, or $y2 = 0.775x + 5.05$.

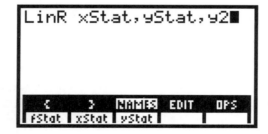

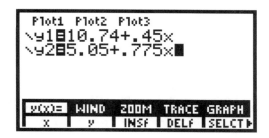

(e) To estimate the year in which the number of U. S. travelers to Europe will be the same as the number of U. S. travelers to Canada, we solve the system of equations

$$y = 0.45x + 10.74,$$
$$y = 0.775x + 5.05.$$

We graph the equations in the same viewing window and then use the Intersect feature to find their point of intersection. Through a trial-and-error process we find that $[0, 25, 0, 25]$ provides a good window in which to see this point.

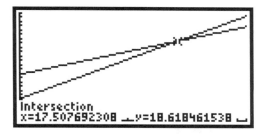

We see that the solution of the system of equations is approximately $(17.51, 18.62)$, so the number of U. S. travelers to Europe will be the same as the number of U. S. travelers to Canada about 17.51 yr after 1990, or in 2008.

ELIMINATION USING MATRICES

Matrices with up to 255 rows or columns can be entered on the TI-86. The row-equivalent operations necessary to write a matrix in row-echelon form or reduced row-echelon form can be performed on the calculator, or we can go directly to either of these forms with a single command. We will illustrate the direct approach for finding reduced row-echelon form.

Section 3.6, Example 4 Solve the following system using a graphing calculator:

$$2x + 5y - 8z = 7,$$
$$3x + 4y - 3z = 8,$$
$$5y - 2x = 9.$$

First we rewrite the third equation in the form $ax + by + cz = d$:

$$2x + 5y - 8z = 7,$$
$$3x + 4y - 3z = 8,$$
$$-2x + 5y \quad\quad = 9.$$

Then we enter the coefficient matrix

$$\begin{bmatrix} 2 & 5 & -8 & 7 \\ 3 & 4 & -3 & 8 \\ -2 & 5 & 0 & 9 \end{bmatrix}$$

in the calculator. Press $\boxed{\text{2nd}}$ $\boxed{\text{MATRX}}$ $\boxed{\text{F2}}$ to display the MATRIX EDIT screen. (MATRX is the second operation associated with the 7 numeric key.) The calculator is now in alphabetic mode, so we press $\boxed{\text{A}}$ to name the matrix "A." (A is the alphabetic operation associated with the $\boxed{\text{LOG}}$ key.) If other matrices have already been named, their names will appear at the bottom of the screen and can be chosen by pressing the $\boxed{\text{F1}}$ - $\boxed{\text{F5}}$ keys. Now press $\boxed{\text{ENTER}}$ to display the matrix editor. The dimensions of the matrix are displayed on the top line of this screen, with the cursor on the row dimension. Enter the dimensions of the coefficient matrix, 3 x 4, by pressing 3 $\boxed{\text{ENTER}}$ 4 $\boxed{\text{ENTER}}$. Now the cursor moves to the element in the first row and first column of the matrix. Enter the elements of the first row by pressing 2 $\boxed{\text{ENTER}}$ 5 $\boxed{\text{ENTER}}$ $\boxed{(-)}$ 8 $\boxed{\text{ENTER}}$ 7 $\boxed{\text{ENTER}}$. The cursor moves to the element in the second row and first column of the matrix. Enter the elements of the second and third rows of the augmented matrix by typing each in turn followed by $\boxed{\text{ENTER}}$ as above. Note that the screen only displays three columns of the matrix. The arrow keys can be used to move the cursor to any element at any time.

Matrix operations are found on the MATRIX OPS menu and are performed on the home screen. Press $\boxed{\text{2nd}}$ $\boxed{\text{QUIT}}$ leave the matrix editor and go to this screen. Then press $\boxed{\text{2nd}}$ $\boxed{\text{MATRX}}$ $\boxed{\text{F4}}$ to access the MATRIX OPS menu. The reduced row-echelon from command is item $\boxed{\text{F5}}$ "rref" on the menu. Copy it to the home screen by pressing $\boxed{\text{F5}}$. We see the command "rref."

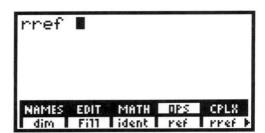

Since we want to find reduced row-echelon form for matrix A, we enter A by pressing $\boxed{\text{ALPHA}}$ $\boxed{\text{A}}$. Alternatively, press $\boxed{\text{2nd}}$ $\boxed{\text{F1}}$ to see the list of names. Then choose A by pressing the key $\boxed{\text{F1}}$ - $\boxed{\text{F5}}$ corresponding to A. To see the elements of the row-echelon form of the matrix in fraction form, press $\boxed{\text{2nd}}$ $\boxed{\text{MATH}}$ $\boxed{\text{F5}}$ $\boxed{\text{MORE}}$ $\boxed{\text{F1}}$. Finally press $\boxed{\text{ENTER}}$ to see this matrix. We see that the solution of the system of equations is $\left(\frac{1}{2}, 2, \frac{1}{2}\right)$.

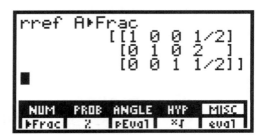

Chapter 4
Inequalities and Problem Solving

GRAPHICAL SOLUTIONS OF INEQUALITIES

Solving inequalities graphically involves first finding a point of intersection.

Section 4.1, Example 4 Solve graphically: $16 - 7x \geq 10x - 4$.

Graph $y_1 = 16 - 7x$ and $y_2 = 10x - 4$ in the window $[-5, 5, -5, 15]$ and find the first coordinate of their point of intersection. It is approximately 1.1764706.

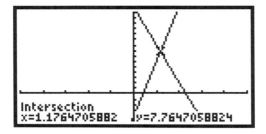

Observe that y_1 (on the graph that slants down from left to right) is greater than y_2 (on the graph that slants up from left to right) to the left of the point of intersection and $y_1 < y_2$ to the right of this point. Thus, the solution set will consist of all x-values to the left of 1.1764706 and also the value 1.1764706 itself since the inequality symbol is $\geq$, or $(-\infty, 1.1764706]$.

Another method for solving inequalities on a graphing calculator makes use of the $\boxed{\text{CATLG-VARS}}$ and $\boxed{\text{TEST}}$ keys. To solve the inequality above this way, we begin as before by finding the first coordinate of the point of intersection of y_1 and y_2. Then return to the equation-editor screen and enter $y_3 = y_1 \geq y_2$ by first positioning the cursor beside $y3 =$ and pressing $\boxed{\text{2nd}}$ $\boxed{\text{CATLG-VARS}}$ $\boxed{\text{MORE}}$ $\boxed{\text{F4}}$. Select $y1$ by positioning the triangular selection cursor beside it and pressing $\boxed{\text{ENTER}}$. Then press $\boxed{\text{2nd}}$ $\boxed{\text{TEST}}$ $\boxed{\text{F5}}$ $\boxed{\text{2nd}}$ $\boxed{\text{CATLG-VARS}}$ $\boxed{\text{MORE}}$ $\boxed{\text{F4}}$. Select $y2$ by positioning the triangular marker beside it and pressing $\boxed{\text{ENTER}}$. (TEST is the second operation associated with the 2 numeric key.) The keystrokes $\boxed{\text{2nd}}$ $\boxed{\text{TEST}}$ $\boxed{\text{F5}}$ display the TEST menu and paste the symbol "$\geq$" from that menu to the equation-editor screen, and the last four keystrokes enter $y2$ after $\geq$.

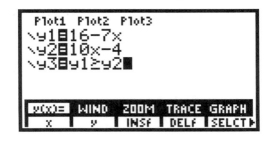

The value of y_3 will be 1 where $y_1 \geq y_2$ is true, and it will be 0 where $y_1 \geq y_2$ is false. Press $\boxed{\text{2nd}}$ $\boxed{\text{F5}}$ to see the graphs of y_1, y_2, and y_3. We use the same window as above.

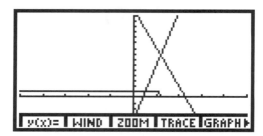

The solution set of $y_1 \geq y_2$ is displayed as an interval shown by a horizontal line 1 unit above the x-axis. The endpoint of this interval corresponds to the first coordinate of the point of intersection of y_1 and y_2. Thus, we see again that the solution set of the original inequality is approximately $(-\infty, 1.1764706]$.

INEQUALITIES IN TWO VARIABLES

The solution set of an inequality in two variables can be graphed on the TI-86.

Section 4.4, Example 4 Use a graphing calculator to graph the inequality $8x + 3y > 24$.

First we write the related equation, $8x + 3y = 24$, and solve it for y. We get $y = -\frac{8}{3}x + 8$. We will enter this as $y1$. Press $\boxed{\text{GRAPH}}$ $\boxed{\text{F1}}$ to go to the equation-editor screen. If there is currently an entry for $y1$, clear it. Also clear or deselect any other equations that are entered and turn off the Plots. Now enter $y_1 = (-8/3)x + 8$. Since the inequality states that $8x + 3y > 24$, or y is *greater than* $-\frac{8}{3}x + 8$, we want to shade the half-plane above the graph of y_1. To do this, first press $\boxed{\text{MORE}}$. The choice "Style" appears above $\boxed{\text{F3}}$. Press $\boxed{\text{F3}}$ until the "shade above" Style icon appears to the left of $y1 =$. If the "line" Style was previously selected, the "Shade above" icon will appear after $\boxed{\text{F3}}$ is pressed two times. (To shade below a line we would press $\boxed{\text{F3}}$ until the "shade below" Style symbol appears.) Then press $\boxed{\text{2nd}}$ $\boxed{\text{F3}}$ $\boxed{\text{F4}}$ to see the graph of the inequality in the standard viewing window.

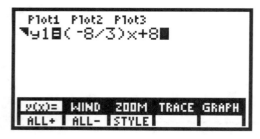
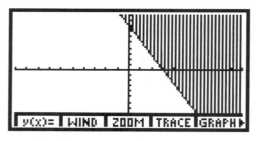

Note that when the "shade above" Style is selected it is not also possible to select the dotted Style so we must keep in mind the fact that the line $y = -\frac{8}{3}x + 8$ is not included in the graph of the inequality. If you graphed this inequality by hand, you would draw a dashed line.

SYSTEMS OF LINEAR INEQUALITIES

We can graph systems of inequalities by shading the solution set of each inequality in the system with a different pattern. When the "shade above" or "shade below" Style options are selected the calculator rotates through four shading patterns. Vertical lines shade the first function, horizontal lines the second, negatively sloping diagonal lines the third, and positively sloping diagonal lines the fourth. These patterns repeat if more than four functions are graphed.

Section 4.4, Example 8 Graph the system

$$x + y \leq 4,$$

$$x - y < 4.$$

First graph the equation $x + y = 4$, entering it in the form $y = -x + 4$. We determine that the solution set of $x + y \leq 4$ consists of all points on or below the line $x + y = 4$, or $y = -x + 4$, so we select the "shade below" Style for this function. Next graph $x - y = 4$, entering it in the form $y = x - 4$. The solution set of $x - y < 4$ is all points above the line $x - y = 4$, or $y = x - 4$, so for this function we choose the "shade above" Style. (See page 84 of this manual for instructions on selecting Style icons.) Now press $\boxed{\text{2nd}}$ $\boxed{\text{F3}}$ $\boxed{\text{F4}}$ to display the solution sets of each inequality in the system and the region where they overlap in the standard viewing window. The region of overlap is the solution set of the system of inequalities. Keep in mind that the line $x + y = 4$, or $y = -x + 4$, is part of the solution set while $x - y = 4$, or $y = x - 4$, is not.

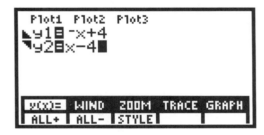   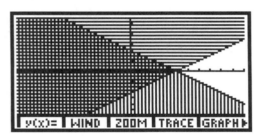

Chapter 5
Polynomials and Polynomial Functions

EVALUATING A POLYNOMIAL FUNCTION

We can use a table set in Ask mode to evaluate a polynomial function.

Section 5.1, Example 4 Find $P(-5)$ for the polynomial function given by $P(x) = -x^2 + 4x - 1$.

To use a table to find this function value, first enter $y1 = -x^2 + 4x - 1$ on the equation-editor screen. Then press $\boxed{\text{TABLE}}$ $\boxed{\text{F2}}$ to display the table set-up screen. To set up a table in which you choose the x-values that are entered, set "Indpnt" to "Ask" by positioning the cursor over "Ask" and pressing $\boxed{\text{ENTER}}$. In Ask mode the calculator disregards the setting of TblStart and ΔTbl.

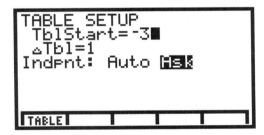

Now press $\boxed{\text{F1}}$ to view the table. Values for x can be entered in the x-column of the table and the corresponding y-values will be displayed in the $y1$-column. To enter -5 for x, press $\boxed{\text{(−)}}$ 5 $\boxed{\text{ENTER}}$. We see that $P(-5) = -46$.

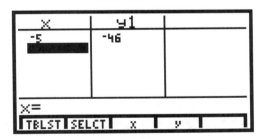

CHECKING OPERATIONS ON POLYNOMIALS

A graphing calculator can be used to check operations on polynomials.

Section 5.1, Example 9 Add: $(-3x^3 + 2x - 4) + (4x^3 + 3x^2 + 2)$.

This addition is carried out in the text, and the result is $x^3 + 3x^2 + 2x - 2$. There are several ways in which we can use a graphing calculator to check this result. One of these is to compare the graphs of $y1 = (-3x^3 + 2x - 4) + (4x^3 + 3x^2 + 2)$ and $y2 = x^3 + 3x^2 + 2x - 2$. This is most easily done when different graph styles are used for the graphs.

Seven graph styles can be selected on the equation-editor screen of the TI-86. The **path graph style** can be used, along with the line style, to determine whether graphs coincide. To use graphs to check the addition in Example 9, first press $\boxed{\text{GRAPH}}$ $\boxed{\text{MORE}}$ $\boxed{\text{F3}}$ to determine whether Sequential graph format is selected. If it is not, position the blinking cursor over SeqG and then press $\boxed{\text{ENTER}}$. Next, on the equation-editor screen, enter $y1 = (-3x^3 + 2x - 4) + (4x^3 + 3x^2 + 2)$ and $y2 = x^3 + 3x^2 + 2x - 2$. We will select the line graph style for $y1$ and the path style for $y2$. To select these graph styles use $\boxed{\triangleleft}$ to position the cursor anywhere in the equation and then press $\boxed{\text{MORE}}$. Now press $\boxed{\text{F3}}$ repeatedly until the desired style icon appears as shown on the right below.

 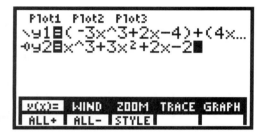

The calculator will graph $y1$ first as a solid line. Then $y2$ will be graphed as the circular cursor traces the leading edge of the graph, allowing us to determine visually whether the graphs coincide. In this case, the graphs appear to coincide, so the factorization is probably correct.

We can also check the addition by **subtracting** the result from the original sum. With $y1$ and $y2$ entered as described above, position the cursor beside "$y3 =$" and use the CATLG-VARS menu to enter $y3 = y1 - y2$. First press $\boxed{\text{2nd}}$ $\boxed{\text{CATLG-VARS}}$ $\boxed{\text{MORE}}$ $\boxed{\text{F4}}$. Position the triangular cursor beside $y1$ and press $\boxed{\text{ENTER}}$. Then press $\boxed{-}$ $\boxed{\text{2nd}}$ $\boxed{\text{CATLG-VARS}}$ $\boxed{\text{MORE}}$ $\boxed{\text{F4}}$. Now position the triangular cursor beside $y2$ and press $\boxed{\text{ENTER}}$.

If the subtraction is correct, $y1 = y2$, so $y3 = 0$. Since we are interested only in the values of $y3$, we deselect $y1$ and $y2$ as described on page 75 of this manual. Select the path style for $y3$ as described above.

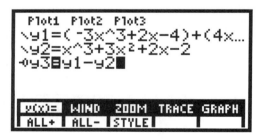

Now press $\boxed{\text{2nd}}$ $\boxed{\text{F5}}$ and determine if the graph of $y3$ is traced over the x-axis. Since it is, the sum is correct.

We can use a table of values to **compare values** of $y1$ and $y2$. If the expressions for $y1$ and $y2$ are the same for each given x-value, the result checks. If you deselected $y1$ and $y2$ to check the sum using subtraction as described above, select them again now. Then look at a table set in Auto mode. Since the values of $y1$ and $y2$ are the same for each given x-value, the result checks. Scrolling through the table to look at additional values makes this conclusion more certain.

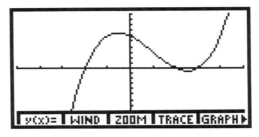

The TI-86 does not have a split screen feature that allows us to view a graph and a table of values simultaneously.

FINDING THE ZEROS OF A FUNCTION

We can use the Root feature from the GRAPH MATH menu to find the zeros of a function. (Sometimes the words "zero" and "root" are used interchangeably, although we make a distinction between them in the text.)

Section 5.3, Example 2 Find the zeros of the function given by $f(x) = x^3 - 3x^2 - 4x + 12$.

First we graph the function in a viewing window that shows the x-intercepts clearly. Through a trial-and-error process we find that $[-5, 5, -20, 20]$, Yscl $= 2$, is a good choice. We see that the function has three zeros. They appear to be about -2, 2, and 3.

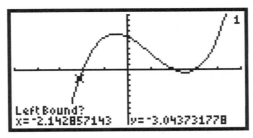

We will find the zero near -2 first. From the GRAPH screen press $\boxed{\text{MORE}}$ $\boxed{\text{F1}}$ $\boxed{\text{F1}}$ to select the Root feature from the GRAPH MATH menu. We are prompted to select a left bound. This means that we must choose an x-value that is to the left of -2 on the x-axis. This can be done by using the left- and right-hand arrow keys to move to a point on the curve to the left of -2 or by keying in a value less than -2.

Once this is done, press $\boxed{\text{ENTER}}$. Now we are prompted to select a right bound that is to the right of -2 on the x-axis. Again, this can be done by using the arrow keys to move to a point on the curve to the right of -2 or by keying in a value greater than -2.

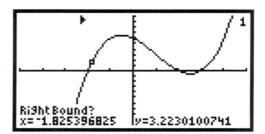

Press $\boxed{\text{ENTER}}$ again. Finally we are prompted to make a guess as to the value of the zero. Move the cursor to a point close to the zero or key in a value.

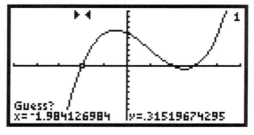

Press $\boxed{\text{ENTER}}$ a third time. We see that $y = 0$ when $x = -2$, so -2 is a zero of the function f.

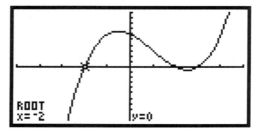

Select Root from the GRAPH MATH menu a second time to find the zero near 2 and a third time to find the zero near 3. We see that the other two zeros are exactly 2 and 3.

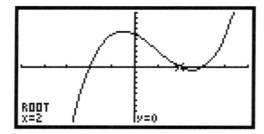
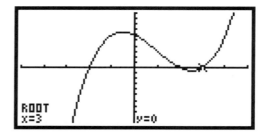

POLYNOMIAL REGRESSION

The TI-86 has the capability to use regression to fit nonlinear polynomial equations to data.

Section 5.8, Example 4(a) The number of bachelor's degrees earned in the biological and life sciences for various years is shown in the following table. Fit a polynomial function of degree 3 (cubic) to the data.

Year	Number of Bachelor's Degrees Earned in Biological/Life Science
1971	35,743
1976	54,275
1980	46,370
1986	38,524
1990	37,204
1994	51,383
2000	63,532

First enter the data with the number of years since 1970 in xStat and the number of bachelor's degrees earned, in thousands, in yStat. (See page 67 of this manual for the procedure to follow.) We select cubic regression, denoted P3Reg, from the STAT CALC menu. Press $\boxed{\text{2nd}}$ $\boxed{\text{QUIT}}$ to go to the home screen. Then press $\boxed{\text{2nd}}$ $\boxed{\text{STAT}}$ $\boxed{\text{F1}}$ $\boxed{\text{MORE}}$ $\boxed{\text{F5}}$ $\boxed{\text{2nd}}$ $\boxed{\text{LIST}}$ $\boxed{\text{F3}}$ $\boxed{\text{F2}}$ $\boxed{,}$ $\boxed{\text{F3}}$ $\boxed{,}$ $\boxed{\text{2nd}}$ $\boxed{\text{ALPHA}}$ $\boxed{\text{Y}}$ $\boxed{1}$ $\boxed{\text{ENTER}}$. These keystrokes instruct the calculator to find the regression equation and to copy it to the equation-editor screen as $y1$. The calculator returns the number of data points along with the coefficients for a cubic function of the form $f(x) = ax^3 + bx^2 + cx + d$. Note that we must use the $\boxed{\triangleright}$ key to scroll across the screen to see all of the coefficients. Rounding the coefficients to the nearest thousandth, we have $f(x) = 0.009x^3 - 0.371x^2 + 4.176x + 34.415$.

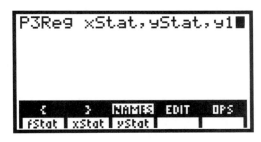 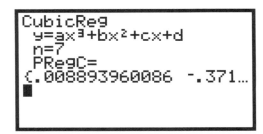

We can use methods discussed earlier in this manual to estimate and predict function values and to find the year or years in which a specific function value occurs.

Chapter 6
Rational Equations and Functions

GRAPHING IN DOT MODE

Consider the graph of the function $T(t) = \dfrac{t^2 + 5t}{2t + 5}$ in Section 6.1, Example 1. Enter $y = (x^2 + 5x)/(2x + 5)$ and graph it in the window $[-5, 5, -5, 5]$.

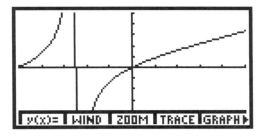

Note that a vertical line that is not part of the graph appears on the screen along with the two branches of the graph. The reason for this is discussed in the text.

This line will not appear if we change from DrawLine format to Dot format. Access the Format screen from the Graph screen by pressing $\boxed{\text{MORE}}$ $\boxed{\text{F3}}$. Then move the cursor to DrawDot on the third line and press $\boxed{\text{ENTER}}$. Now press $\boxed{\text{F5}}$ to see the graph of the function in Dot format.

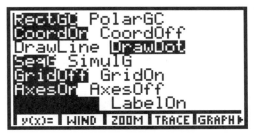 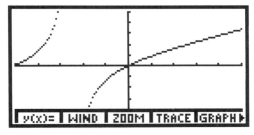

We can also select Dot format by selecting the "dot" Style on the equation-editor screen. If the function $T(t) = \dfrac{t^2 + 5t}{2t + 5}$ is entered as $y_1 = (x^2 + 5x)/(2x + 5)$, for instance, position the cursor beside $y_1 =$, press $\boxed{\text{MORE}}$, and then press $\boxed{\text{F3}}$ repeatedly until the "dot" icon appears. If the "line" icon was previously selected, $\boxed{\text{F3}}$ must be pressed six times to select the "dot" style.

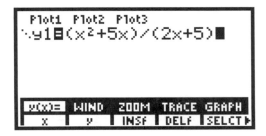

Chapter 7
Exponents and Radical Functions

RADICAL EXPRESSIONS AND RATIONAL EXPONENTS

As discussed in Section 7.2, we can enter a radical expression using radical notation or rational exponents. For example, we can enter $y = \sqrt{x-3}$ using radical notation or as $y = (x-2)^{1/2}$ or as $y = (x-3)^{0.5}$. To enter $= \sqrt{x-3}$, press $\boxed{\text{2nd}}$ $\boxed{\sqrt{}}$ $\boxed{(}$ $\boxed{\text{x-VAR}}$ $\boxed{-}$ 3 $\boxed{)}$. ($\sqrt{}$ is the second operation associated with the $\boxed{x^2}$ key.) Note that, since the radicand has more than one term, we must enclose it in parentheses. To enter $y = (x-3)^{1/2}$, press $\boxed{(}$ $\boxed{\text{x-VAR}}$ $\boxed{-}$ 3 $\boxed{)}$ $\boxed{\wedge}$ $\boxed{(}$ 1 $\boxed{\div}$ 2 $\boxed{)}$. Note that both the radicand and the rational exponent are enclosed in parentheses. To enter $y = (x-3)^{0.5}$, press $\boxed{(}$ $\boxed{\text{X, T, } \Theta, n}$ $\boxed{-}$ 3 $\boxed{)}$ $\boxed{\wedge}$ 0 $\boxed{\cdot}$ 5. When the exponent is in decimal notation it is not necessary to enclose it in parentheses.

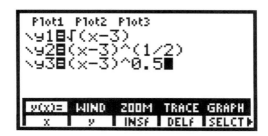

We can use either the xth root option from the MATH MISC menu or a rational exponent to enter a cube root. For example, to enter $y = \sqrt[3]{x+5}$ using radical notation first enter the index of the radical, 3. Then select the xth root option and finally enter the radicand enclosed in parentheses. To do this, press 3 $\boxed{\text{2nd}}$ $\boxed{\text{MATH}}$ $\boxed{\text{F5}}$ $\boxed{\text{MORE}}$ $\boxed{\text{F4}}$ $\boxed{(}$ $\boxed{\text{x-VAR}}$ $\boxed{+}$ 5 $\boxed{)}$. The keystrokes $\boxed{\text{2nd}}$ $\boxed{\text{MATH}}$ $\boxed{\text{F5}}$ $\boxed{\text{MORE}}$ $\boxed{\text{F4}}$ access the MATH MISC menu and then select the xth root option from that menu. Using a rational exponent, we can enter $y = \sqrt[3]{x+5}$ as $y = (x+5)^{1/3}$. Press $\boxed{(}$ $\boxed{\text{x-VAR}}$ $\boxed{+}$ 5 $\boxed{)}$ $\boxed{\wedge}$ $\boxed{(}$ 1 $\boxed{\div}$ 3 $\boxed{)}$. Since we cannot enter exact decimal notation for 1/3, we cannot use decimal notation for the exponent in this case.

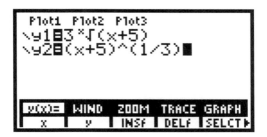

To enter $f(x) = \sqrt[4]{2x-7}$, as in Section 7.2, Example 3, we also use the xth root option from the MATH MISC menu. To do this we first enter the index of the radical, 4. Then select the xth root feature and, finally, enter the radicand, $2x-7$. Press 4 $\boxed{\text{2nd}}$ $\boxed{\text{MATH}}$ $\boxed{\text{F5}}$ $\boxed{\text{MORE}}$ $\boxed{\text{F4}}$ $\boxed{(}$ 2 $\boxed{\text{X, T, } \Theta, n}$ $\boxed{-}$ 7 $\boxed{)}$. We could also enter this function as $f(x) = (2x-7)^{1/4}$ or as

$f(x) = (2x - 7)^{0.25}$.

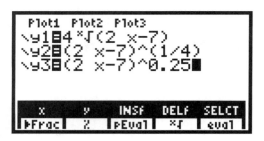

Chapter 8
Quadratic Functions and Equations

FINDING THE VERTEX

We can use a graphing calculator to find the vertex of a quadratic function. We do this by using the Maximum or Minimum feature from the GRAPH MATH menu.

Section 8.7, Example 4 Use a graphing calculator to determine the vertex of the graph of the function given by $f(x) = -2x^2 + 10x - 7$.

The coefficient of x^2 is negative, so we know that the graph of the function opens down and, thus, has a maximum value. Clear or deselect any functions previously entered on the equation-editor screen. Then enter $y = -2x^2 + 10x - 7$. Choose a viewing window that shows the vertex. One good choice is $[-3, 7, -10, 10]$.

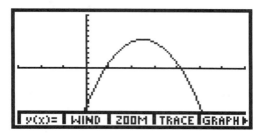

Now select the Maximum feature from the GRAPH MATH menu by pressing $\boxed{\text{MORE}}$ $\boxed{\text{F1}}$ $\boxed{\text{F5}}$. We are prompted to select a left bound for the vertex. Use the arrow keys to move the cursor to a point on the parabola to the left of the vertex or key in an x-value that is less than the x-coordinate of the vertex.

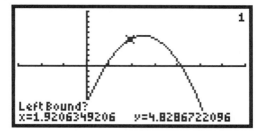

Press $\boxed{\text{ENTER}}$. Next we are prompted to select a right bound. Move the cursor to a point on the parabola to the right of the vertex or key in an x-value that is greater than the x-coordinate of the vertex.

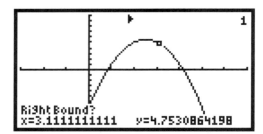

Press ENTER . We are now prompted to make a guess as to the x-coordinate of the vertex. Move the cursor close to the vertex or key in an x-value close to the x-value of the vertex.

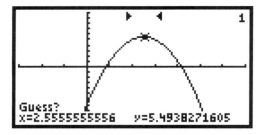

Press ENTER a third time. We see that the maximum function value is 5.5, and it occurs when x is approximately 2.5. Thus, the vertex of the graph of $f(x) = -2x^2 + 10x97$ is $(2.5, 5.5)$. (Note that, because of the method the calculator uses to find the maximum function value, the coordinates might not be exact and can vary slightly depending on the window chosen.)

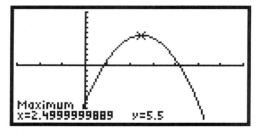

Minimum function values are found in a similar manner. From the Graph screen, select the Minimum feature from the GRAPH MATH menu by pressing MORE F1 F4 .

QUADRATIC REGRESSION

Regression can be used to fit a quadratic function to data when three or more data points are given.

Section 8.8, Example 4(c) According to the Centers for Disease Control and Prevention, the percent of high school students who reported having smoked a cigarette in the preceding 30 days declined from 1997 to 2001, after rising in the first part of the 1990s. Use the REGRESSION feature of a graphing calculator to fit a quadratic function $H(x)$ to all the given data in the following table.

Years after 1991	Percent of High School Students Who Smoked a Cigarette in the Preceding 30 Days
0	27.5
2	30.5
4	34.9
6	36.4
8	34.9
10	28.5

We enter the data in xStat and yStat as described on page 67 of this manual.

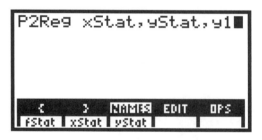

Then press 2nd QUIT to go to the home screen and select P2Reg from the STAT CALC menu by pressing 2nd STAT F1 MORE F4 2nd LIST F3 F2 , F3 , 2nd alpha Y 1 ENTER . The calculator returns the coefficients of a quadratic function $y = ax^2 + bx + c$ and copies the function to the equation-editor screen as y1. We have $H(x) = -0.315178571429x^2 + 3.43321628571x + 26.5071428571$.

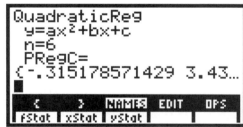

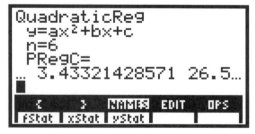

The function can be evaluated using one of the methods on pages 71 and 72 of this manual.

Chapter 9
Exponential and Logarithmic Functions

COMPOSITE FUNCTIONS

For functions y_1 and y_2, when we enter $y_1(y_2)$ on a graphing calculator we are entering the composition $y_1 \circ y_2$. The composite functions found in Section 9.1, Example 2 are checked using tables on a graphing calculator. To check that $f \circ g = \sqrt{x-1}$ when $f(x) = \sqrt{x}$ and $g(x) = x - 1$, enter $y_1 = \sqrt{x}$, $y_2 = x - 1$, $y_3 = \sqrt{x-1}$, and $y_4 = y_1(y_2)$ on the equation-editor screen. To enter $y4$, position the cursor beside $y4 =$ and press $\boxed{\text{F2}}$ 1 $\boxed{(}$ $\boxed{\text{F2}}$ 2 $\boxed{)}$. Then compare the values of y_3 and y_4 in a table. We show a table with TblStart $= 1$, ΔTbl $= 0.5$, and Indpnt and Depend both set on Auto. Use the $\boxed{\triangleright}$ key to scroll across the table to see the y_3- and y_4-columns.

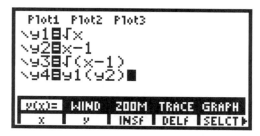

Similarly, to check that $g \circ f(x) = \sqrt{x} - 1$, also enter $y_5 = \sqrt{x} - 1$ and $y_6 = y_2(y_1)$. To enter y_6, position the cursor beside $y6 =$ and press $\boxed{\text{F2}}$ 2 $\boxed{(}$ $\boxed{\text{F2}}$ 1 $\boxed{)}$.

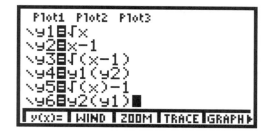

GRAPHING FUNCTIONS AND THEIR INVERSES

We can graph the inverse of a function using the DrInv feature from the DRAW menu.

Section 9.1, Example 9(c) Graph the inverse of the function $g(x) = x^3 + 2$.

We will graph $g(x)$, $g^{-1}(x)$, and the line $y = x$ on the same screen. Press $\boxed{\text{GRAPH}}$ $\boxed{\text{F1}}$ to go to the equation-editor screen and clear or deselect any existing entries. Then enter $y_1 = x^3 + 2$ and $y_2 = x$. Select a square window by pressing $\boxed{\text{2nd}}$ $\boxed{\text{F3}}$ $\boxed{\text{MORE}}$ $\boxed{\text{F2}}$. Now find the DrInv command in the Catalog by pressing $\boxed{\text{2nd}}$ $\boxed{\text{CATLG-VARS}}$ $\boxed{\text{F1}}$ $\boxed{\text{D}}$ and using the $\boxed{\triangledown}$ key to scroll down to DrInv. Copy this command to the home screen by pressing $\boxed{\text{ENTER}}$. Indicate that we want to draw the inverse of y_1 by pressing $\boxed{\text{2nd}}$ $\boxed{\text{alpha}}$ $\boxed{\text{Y}}$ 1. Finally press $\boxed{\text{ENTER}}$ to see the graph of y_1^{-1} along with the graphs of y_1 and y_2. We show a window that has been squared from the standard window.

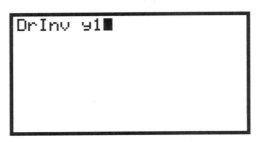   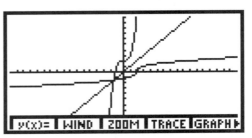

The drawing of y_1^{-1} can be cleared from the graph screen by pressing $\boxed{\text{MORE}}$ $\boxed{\text{F2}}$ $\boxed{\text{MORE}}$ $\boxed{\text{MORE}}$ $\boxed{\text{F1}}$ to select the CLRDRW (clear drawing) operation. CLRDRW can also be accessed from the catalog. If this is done, $\boxed{\text{ENTER}}$ must be pressed after the operation is pasted to the home screen.

GRAPHING LOGARITHMIC FUNCTIONS

Section 9.3, Example 4 Graph: $f(x) = \log \dfrac{x}{5} + 1$.

We enter $y = \log(x/5) + 1$ on the equation-editor screen by positioning the cursor beside one of the function names and pressing $\boxed{\text{LOG}}$ $\boxed{(}$ $\boxed{\text{x-VAR}}$ $\boxed{\div}$ 5 $\boxed{)}$ $\boxed{+}$ 1. Note that the fraction must be entered in parentheses. (Clear or deselect any previously entered functions.) We show the function graphed in the window $[-2, 10, -5, 5]$.

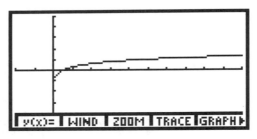

MORE ON GRAPHING

Section 9.5, Example 4 Graph: $f(x) = e^{-0.5x} + 1$.

We enter $y = e^{-0.5x} + 1$ on the equation-editor screen by positioning the cursor beside one of the function names and pressing $\boxed{\text{2nd}}$ $\boxed{e^x}$ $\boxed{(}$ $\boxed{(-)}$. 5 $\boxed{\text{x-VAR}}$ $\boxed{)}$ $\boxed{+}$ 1. (Clear or deselect any previously entered functions.) Select a window and press $\boxed{\text{F5}}$. We show the function graphed in the window $[-5, 5, -2, 10]$.

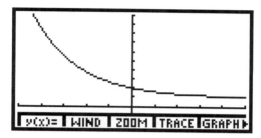

Section 9.5, Example 5(b) Graph: $f(x) = \ln(x + 3)$.

We enter $y = \ln(x + 3)$ on the equation-editor screen by positioning the cursor beside one of the function names and pressing $\boxed{\text{LN}}$ $\boxed{(}$ $\boxed{\text{x-VAR}}$ $\boxed{+}$ 3 $\boxed{)}$. (Clear or deselect any previously entered functions.) Select a window and, from the WINDOW screen, press $\boxed{\text{F5}}$. We show the function graphed in the window $[-5, 10, -5, 5]$.

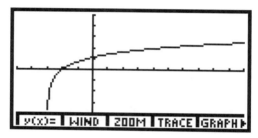

Section 9.5, Example 6 Graph: $f(x) = \log_7 x + 2$.

To use a graphing calculator we must first change the logarithmic base to e or 10. We will use e here. Recall that the change of base formula is $\log_b M = \dfrac{\log_a M}{\log_a b}$, where a and b are any logarithmic bases and M is any positive number. Let $a = e$, $b = 7$, and $M = x$ and substitute in the change-of-base formula. After clearing or deselecting previously entered functions, enter $y_1 = \dfrac{\ln x}{\ln 7} + 2$ on the equation-editor screen by positioning the cursor beside $y1 =$ and pressing $\boxed{\text{LN}}$ $\boxed{\text{x-VAR}}$ $\boxed{\div}$ $\boxed{\text{LN}}$ 7 $\boxed{+}$ 2.

Select a viewing window and press $\boxed{\text{F5}}$. We show the graph in the window $[-2, 8, -2, 5]$.

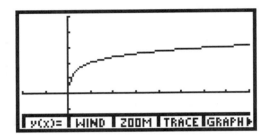

EXPONENTIAL REGRESSION

The STAT CALC menu contains an exponential regression feature.

Section 9.7, Example 9(a) In 1800, over 500,000 Tule elk inhabited the state of California. By the late 1800s, after the California Gold Rush, there were fewer than 50 elk remaining in the state. In 1978, wildlife biologists introduced a herd of 10 Tule elk into the Point Reyes National Seashore near San Francisco. By 1982, the herd had grown to 24 elk. There were 70 elk in 1986, 200 in 1996, and 500 in 2002. Use regression to fit an exponential function to the data and graph the function.

We enter the data as described on page 67 of this manual. Let x represent the number of years since 1978.

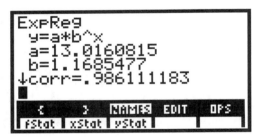

Now press $\boxed{\text{2nd}}$ $\boxed{\text{QUIT}}$ to go to the home screen. Select ExpR from the STAT CALC menu by pressing $\boxed{\text{2nd}}$ $\boxed{\text{F1}}$ $\boxed{\text{F5}}$ $\boxed{\text{2nd}}$ $\boxed{\text{LIST}}$ $\boxed{\text{F3}}$ $\boxed{\text{F2}}$ $\boxed{,}$ $\boxed{\text{F3}}$ $\boxed{\text{ENTER}}$. The calculator returns the values of a and b for the exponential function $y = ab^x$. We have $f(x) = 13.0160815(1.1685477)^x$.

This function can be copied to the equation-editor screen using one of the methods described on pages 76 and 77 of this manual. It can be evaluated using one of the methods on pages 71 and 72.

Chapter 10
Sequences, Series, and the Binomial Theorem

SEQUENCES

Section 10.1, Example 1 Find the first four terms and the 13th term of the sequence for which the general term is given by $a_n = (-1)^n n^2$.

Press ⌷GRAPH⌷ ⌷F1⌷ to go to the equation-editor screen. Then enter the general term of the sequence as $y1 = (-1)^x x^2$ by positioning the cursor beside $y1 =$ and pressing ⌷(⌷ ⌷(-)⌷ ⌷1⌷ ⌷)⌷ ⌷∧⌷ ⌷x-VAR⌷ ⌷×⌷ ⌷x-VAR⌷ ⌷x^2⌷. (Clear or deselect any other previously entered functions.)

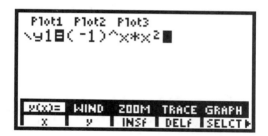

Now set up a table with Indpnt set to Ask. (See page 87 of this manual.) To see the first four terms and the 13th term of the sequence enter 1, 2, 3, 4, and 13 for n in the table.

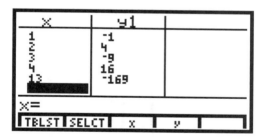

THE SEQUENCE FEATURE

The Sequence feature of the TI-86 writes the terms of a sequence as a list.

Section 10.1, Example 2 Use a graphing calculator to find the first five terms of the sequence for which the general term is given by $a_n = n/(n+1)^2$.

We will copy the Sequence feature from the LIST OPS menu to the home screen by pressing ⌷2nd⌷ ⌷LIST⌷ ⌷F5⌷ ⌷MORE⌷ ⌷F3⌷. Now enter the general term of the sequence, the variable, and the values of the variable for the first and last terms we wish to calculate, all separated by commas. Press ⌷x-VAR⌷ ⌷÷⌷ ⌷(⌷ ⌷x-VAR⌷ ⌷+⌷ ⌷1⌷ ⌷)⌷ ⌷x^2⌷ ⌷,⌷ ⌷x-VAR⌷ ⌷,⌷ ⌷1⌷ ⌷,⌷ ⌷5⌷ ⌷)⌷. We will also choose to display the terms of the sequence as fractions by pressing $\boxed{\text{2nd}}$ $\boxed{\text{MATH}}$ $\boxed{\text{F5}}$ $\boxed{\text{MORE}}$ $\boxed{\text{F1}}$ following the keystrokes shown above. Now press $\boxed{\text{ENTER}}$ to see a list of the first five terms of the sequence. Note that we must use the $\boxed{\triangleright}$ key to see the fifth term in the list.

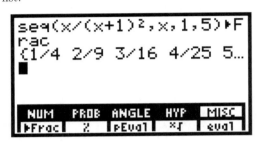 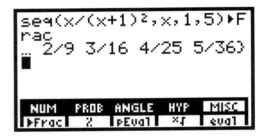

FINDING PARTIAL SUMS

We can use a graphing calculator to find partial sums of a sequence for which the general term is given by a formula.

Section 10.1, Example 5   Use a graphing calculator to find S_1, S_2, S_3, and S_4 for the sequence in which the general term is given by $a_n = (-1)^n/(n+1)$.

We will use the cSum feature from the LIST OPS menu. This option lists the cumulative, or partial, sums for a sequence defined using the Sequence feature discussed above. First copy cSum to the home screen by pressing $\boxed{\text{2nd}}$ $\boxed{\text{LIST}}$ $\boxed{\text{F5}}$ $\boxed{\text{MORE}}$ $\boxed{\text{MORE}}$ $\boxed{\text{F3}}$. Next copy the Sequence feature by pressing $\boxed{\text{2nd}}$ $\boxed{\text{LIST}}$ $\boxed{\text{F5}}$ $\boxed{\text{MORE}}$ $\boxed{\text{F3}}$. Now enter the general term of the sequence, the variable, and the first and last partial sums we wish to calculate, all separated by commas. We will also select the Fraction option from the MATH MISC menu so that the partial sums will be displayed as fractions. Press $\boxed{(}$ $\boxed{(-)}$ $\boxed{1}$ $\boxed{)}$ $\boxed{\wedge}$ $\boxed{\text{x-VAR}}$ $\boxed{\div}$ $\boxed{(}$ $\boxed{\text{x-VAR}}$ $\boxed{+}$ $\boxed{1}$ $\boxed{)}$ $\boxed{,}$ $\boxed{\text{x-VAR}}$ $\boxed{,}$ $\boxed{1}$ $\boxed{,}$ $\boxed{4}$ $\boxed{)}$ $\boxed{)}$ $\boxed{\text{2nd}}$ $\boxed{\text{MATH}}$ $\boxed{\text{F5}}$ $\boxed{\text{MORE}}$ $\boxed{\text{F1}}$ $\boxed{\text{ENTER}}$. Note that we must use the $\boxed{\triangleright}$ key to see S_4.

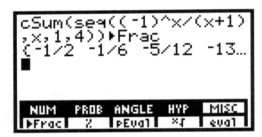 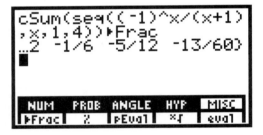

GRAPHING SEQUENCES

The TI-86 does not have a Sequence mode that allows us to graph sequences straightforwardly.

EVALUATING FACTORIALS

Factorials can be evaluated on a graphing calculator.

Section 10.4, Example 3 Simplify: $\dfrac{8!}{5!3!}$.

We use the factorial feature, denoted !, from the MATH PROB (probability) menu. On the home screen press 8 $\boxed{\text{2nd}}$ $\boxed{\text{MATH}}$ $\boxed{\text{F2}}$ $\boxed{\text{F1}}$ $\boxed{\div}$ $\boxed{(}$ 5 $\boxed{\text{F1}}$ 3 $\boxed{\text{F1}}$ $\boxed{)}$ $\boxed{\text{ENTER}}$. Note that we must use parentheses in the denominator so that 8! is divided by both 5! and 3!.

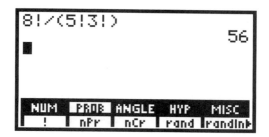

SIMPLIFYING $\left(\begin{smallmatrix} n \\ r \end{smallmatrix} \right)$ NOTATION

Section 10.4, Example 4(a) Simplify: $\left(\begin{smallmatrix} 7 \\ 2 \end{smallmatrix} \right)$.

The calculator uses the notation $_nC_r$ instead of $\left(\begin{smallmatrix} n \\ r \end{smallmatrix} \right)$. This option is found in the MATH PROB menu. To simplify $\left(\begin{smallmatrix} 7 \\ 2 \end{smallmatrix} \right)$, first press 7, then select $_nC_r$ from the MATH PROB menu by pressing $\boxed{\text{2nd}}$ $\boxed{\text{MATH}}$ $\boxed{\text{F2}}$ $\boxed{\text{F3}}$, and then press 2 $\boxed{\text{ENTER}}$.

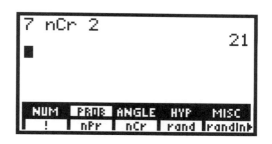

The TI-89
Graphics Calculator

Chapter 1
Basics of Algebra and Graphing

GETTING STARTED

Press $\boxed{\text{ON}}$ to turn on the TI-89 graphing calculator. ($\boxed{\text{ON}}$ is the key at the bottom left-hand corner of the keypad.) The home screen is displayed. You should see a row of boxes at the top of the screen and two horizontal lines with lettering below them at the bottom of the screen. If you do not see anything, try adjusting the display contrast. To do this, first press $\boxed{\diamond}$. ($\boxed{\diamond}$ is the key in the left column of the keypad with a green diamond inside a green border. All operations associated with the $\boxed{\diamond}$ key are printed on the keyboard in green, the same color as the $\boxed{\diamond}$ key.) Then press $\boxed{+}$ to darken the display or $\boxed{-}$ to lighten the display. Be sure to use the black $\boxed{-}$ key in the right column of the keypad rather than the gray $\boxed{(-)}$ key on the bottom row.

One way to turn the calculator off is to press $\boxed{\text{2nd}}$ $\boxed{\text{OFF}}$. (OFF is the second operation associated with the $\boxed{\text{ON}}$ key. All operations accessed by using the $\boxed{\text{2nd}}$ key are printed on the keyboard in yellow, the same color as the $\boxed{\text{2nd}}$ key.) When you turn the TI-89 on again the home screen will be displayed regardless of the screen that was displayed when the calculator was turned off. $\boxed{\text{2nd}}$ $\boxed{\text{OFF}}$ cannot be used to turn off the calculator if an error message is displayed. The calculator can also be turned off by pressing $\boxed{\diamond}$ $\boxed{\text{OFF}}$. This will work even if an error message is displayed. When the TI-89 is turned on again the display will be exactly as it was when it was turned off. The calculator will turn itself off automatically after several minutes without any activity. When this happens the display will be just as you left it when you turn the calculator on again.

From top to bottom, the home screen consists of the toolbar, the large history area where entries and their corresponding results are displayed, the entry line where expressions or instructions are entered, and the status line which shows the current state of the calculator. These areas will be discussed in more detail as the need arises.

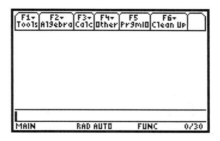

Press $\boxed{\text{MODE}}$ to display the MODE settings. Modes that are not currently valid, due to the existing choices of settings, are dimmed. Initially you should select the settings shown below.

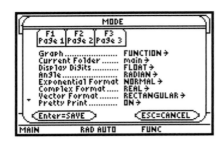
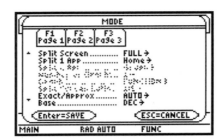

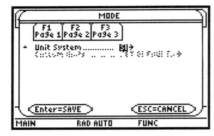

To change a setting on the Mode screen use $\triangledown$ or $\triangle$ to move the cursor to the line of that setting. Then use $\triangleright$ to display the options. Press the number of the desired option followed by ENTER . Press HOME or 2nd QUIT to leave the MODE screen and return to the home screen. (QUIT is the second operation associated with the ESC key.) Note that the cursor skips dimmed settings as you move through the options.

It will be helpful to read the Introduction to the Graphing Calculator on pages 9 and 10 of the textbook as well as Chapter 1: Getting Started and Chapter 2: Operating the TI-89 in the TI-89 Guidebook before proceeding.

ORDER OF OPERATIONS

The TI-89 follows the rules for order of operations.

Section 1.1, Example 9 Evaluate $2(y-3)^2 + 7$ for $y = 5$.

Enter the expression on the entry line of the home screen, substituting 5 for y. You might want to clear any previously entered computations from the history area of the home screen first. To do this, access Tools from the toolbar at the top of the screen by pressing F1 , the blue key at the top left-hand corner of the keypad. Then select item 8, Clear Home, from this menu by pressing 8.

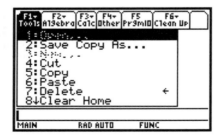

The entry line on the home screen can be cleared by pressing CLEAR . This is not necessary if the current entry is highlighted, since it will automatically be cleared when the first character of a new entry is entered.

Now, to evaluate $2(y-3)^2 + 7$ for $y = 5$, press 2 $\boxed{(}$ 5 $\boxed{-}$ 3 $\boxed{)}$ $\boxed{\wedge}$ 2 $\boxed{+}$ 7 $\boxed{\text{ENTER}}$. Note that the black $\boxed{-}$ key in the right-hand column of the keypad is the subtraction key. The gray $\boxed{(-)}$ key on the bottom row of the keypad represents "the opposite of" or "the additive inverse of" rather than subtraction.

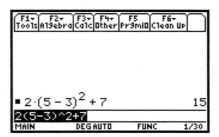

In the expression above we squared $(5-3)$ by pressing $\boxed{\wedge}$ 2. The $\boxed{\wedge}$ key indicates exponentiation and the number following it indicates the exponent. Note that, although the $\wedge$ symbol appears in the expression on the entry line, the history area shows the exponent in the traditional format. This happens because we selected Pretty Print mode earlier.

You can edit your entry if necessary. After $\boxed{\text{ENTER}}$ is pressed to evaluate an expression, the TI-89 leaves the expression on the entry line and highlights it. To edit the expression you must first remove the highlight to avoid the possibility of accidently typing over the entire expression. To do this, press $\boxed{\triangleleft}$ or $\boxed{\triangleright}$ to move the cursor (a blinking vertical line) toward the side of the expression to be edited. If, for instance, in the expression above you pressed 8 instead of 5, first press $\boxed{\triangleleft}$ to move the cursor toward the 8. Now, to type a 5 over the 8, first select overtype mode by pressing $\boxed{\text{2nd}}$ $\boxed{\text{INS}}$. (INS is the second operation associated with the $\boxed{\leftarrow}$ key.) Now the cursor becomes a dark, blinking rectangle rather than a vertical line. Use $\boxed{\triangleright}$ to position the cursor over the 8 and then press 5 to write a 5 over the 8. To leave overtype mode press $\boxed{\text{2nd}}$ $\boxed{\text{INS}}$ again. The calculator is now in the insert mode, indicated by a vertical cursor, and will remain in that mode until overtype mode is once again selected.

If you forgot to type the left parenthesis, move the insert cursor to the left of 5 and press $\boxed{(}$ to insert the parenthesis before the 5. You can continue to insert symbols immediately after the first insertion. If you typed 21 instead of 2, move the cursor to the left of 1 and press $\boxed{\leftarrow}$. This will delete the 1. Instead of using overtype mode to overtype a character as described above, we can use $\boxed{\leftarrow}$ to delete the character and then, in insert mode, insert a new character.

If you accidently press $\boxed{\triangle}$ instead of $\boxed{\triangleleft}$ or $\boxed{\triangleright}$ while editing an expression, the cursor will move up into the history area of the screen. Press $\boxed{\text{ESC}}$ to return immediately to the entry line. The $\boxed{\triangledown}$ key can also be used to return to the entry line. It must be pressed the same number of times the $\boxed{\triangle}$ key was pressed accidently.

If you notice that an entry needs to be edited before you press $\boxed{\text{ENTER}}$ to perform the computation, the editing can be done as described above without the necessity of first removing the highlight from the entry.

The keystrokes $\boxed{\text{2nd}}$ $\boxed{\text{ENTRY}}$ can be used repeatedly to recall entries preceding the last one. (ENTRY is the second function associated with the $\boxed{\text{ENTER}}$ key.) Pressing $\boxed{\text{2nd}}$ $\boxed{\text{ENTRY}}$ twice, for example, will recall the next to last entry. Using these keystrokes a third time recalls the third to last entry and so on. The number of entries that can be recalled depends on the amount of storage they occupy in the calculator's memory.

Previous entries and results of computations can also be copied to the entry line by first using the $\triangle$ key to move through the history area until the desired entry or result is highlighted. Then press ENTER to copy it to the entry line.

USING A MENU

In the previous example we used the Tools menu to clear the home screen.

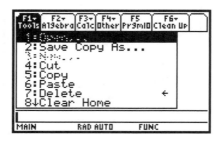

In general, a menu is a list of options that appear when a key is pressed. For example, we pressed F1 to display the Tools menu. We can select an item from a menu by using $\triangledown$ to highlight it and then pressing ENTER or by simply pressing the number of the item. If an item is identified by a letter rather than a number, press the purple alpha key followed by the letter of the item. The letters are printed in purple above the keys on the keypad. The down-arrow beside item 8 in the menu above indicates that there are additional items in the menu. Use $\triangledown$ to scroll down to them.

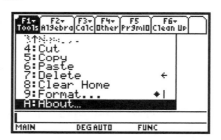

Section 1.2, Example 13 Calculate: $\dfrac{14 - 3| - 16 + 38|}{4| - 2^4 - 3^2|}$.

In order to divide the entire numerator of this fraction by the entire denominator, we must enclose both the numerator and the denominator in parentheses. Recall also that the gray $(-)$ key in the bottom row of the keypad must be used to enter a negative number on the calculator whereas the black $-$ key is used to enter subtraction. On the TI-89, $|x|$ is written abs(x). Absolute value notation is the first item in the calculator's catalog, an alphabetic list of all the commands on the TI-89.

To enter the expression above, go to the entry line of the home screen and press (1 4 $-$ 3 CATALOG A ENTER $(-)$ 1 6 $+$ 3 8)) $\div$ (4 CATALOG ENTER $(-)$ 2 $\wedge$ 4 $-$ 3 $\wedge$ 2)) ENTER. If the triangular selection cursor is already positioned beside abs in the catalog, it is not necessary to include A is the keystrokes above.

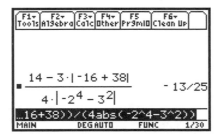

Observe that the calculator supplies the left parenthesis in the absolute value notation. The absolute value expression must be closed with a right parenthesis which must be entered manually. The second right parenthesis in the numerator serves, along with the first left parenthesis, to enclose the entire numerator in parentheses. This is done in the denominator as well.

Note that the result of the calculation above was expressed in fractional notation. This will occur when Exact is selected as the Exact/Approx mode on the Mode screen. It will also occur when the Auto setting is selected and there is no decimal point in the entry.

To see the result expressed in decimal notation, we can enter the expression as above and then press $\boxed{\diamond}$ before pressing $\boxed{\text{ENTER}}$. Note the black $\diamond$ at the bottom of the screen on the left below and the decimal result on the right.

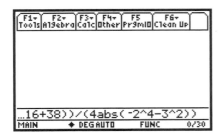 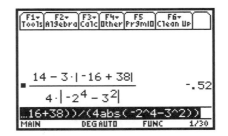

We will also see the result expressed in decimal notation if Approximate is selected as the Exact/Approx mode before entering the expression.

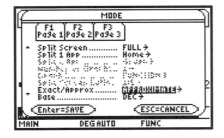 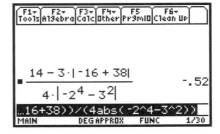

In addition, with Auto mode selected, the result will be expressed in decimal notation if we include a decimal point with one of the integers in the expressions. If we enter $\dfrac{14. - 3|-16+38|}{4|-2^4-3^2|}$ in Auto mode, for example, the result is -0.52.

To convert a fractional result to decimal form, use $\boxed{\triangle}$ to move into the history area and highlight the result. Press $\boxed{\text{ENTER}}$ to copy the result to the entry line. Then press $\boxed{\diamond}$ $\boxed{\text{ENTER}}$ to see the decimal form of the result. This occurs regardless of the Exact/Approx setting. (Note that we ordinarily set the calculator in Auto mode.)

SCIENTIFIC NOTATION

To enter a number in scientific notation, first type the decimal portion of the number; then press the $\boxed{\text{EE}}$ key in the left column of the keypad; finally type the exponent, which can be at most three digits. For example, to enter 1.789×10^{-11} in scientific notation, press $1\ \boxed{.}\ 7\ 8\ 9\ \boxed{\text{EE}}\ \boxed{(-)}\ 1\ 1\ \boxed{\text{ENTER}}$. To enter 6.084×10^{23} in scientific notation, press $6\ \boxed{.}\ 0\ 8\ 4\ \boxed{\text{EE}}\ 2\ 3\ \boxed{\text{ENTER}}$. The decimal portion of each number appears before a small E while the exponent follows the E.

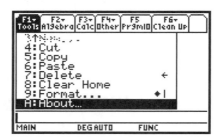

The TI-89 can be used to perform computations in scientific notation.

Section 1.4, Example 14 Use a graphing calculator to check the computation $(7.2 \times 10^5)(4.3 \times 10^9) = 3.096 \times 10^{15}$.

We enter the computation in scientific notation on the entry line of the home screen. Press $7\ \boxed{.}\ 2\ \boxed{\text{EE}}\ 5\ \boxed{\times}\ 4\ \boxed{.}\ 3\ \boxed{\text{EE}}\ 9$ $\boxed{\text{ENTER}}$. We have 3.096×10^{15}, which checks.

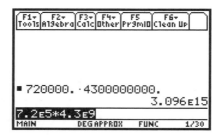

SETTING THE VIEWING WINDOW

The viewing window is the portion of the coordinate plane that appears on the graphing calculator's screen. It is defined by the minimum and maximum values of x and y: xmin, xmax, ymin, and ymax. The notation [xmin, xmax, ymin, ymax] is used in the text to represent these window settings or dimensions. For example, $[-12, 12, -8, 8]$ denotes a window that displays the portion of the x-axis from -12 to 12 and the portion of the y-axis from -8 to 8. In addition, the distance between tick marks on the axes is defined by the settings xscl and yscl. In this manual xscl and yscl will be assumed to be 1 unless noted otherwise. The setting xres sets the pixel resolution. We usually select xres = 2. The window corresponding to the settings $[-20, 30, -12, 20]$, xscl = 5, yscl = 2, xres = 2, is shown below.

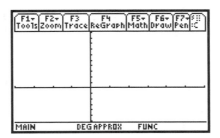

Press [◇] [WINDOW] to display the current window settings on your calculator. (WINDOW is the ◇ operation associated with the [F2] key on the top row of the keypad.) The standard settings are shown below.

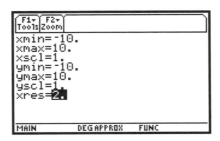

To change a setting, position the cursor beside the setting you wish to change and enter the new value. For example, to change from the standard settings to [−20, 30, −12, 20], xscl = 5, yscl = 2, on the Window screen, start with the setting beside xmin = highlighted and press [(−)] 2 0 [ENTER] 3 0 [ENTER] 5 [ENTER] [(−)] 1 2 [ENTER] 2 0 [ENTER] 2 [ENTER]. The [▽] key may be used instead of [ENTER] after typing each window setting. To see the window shown on the previous page, press [◇] [GRAPH]. (GRAPH is the ◇ operation associated with the [F3] key on the top row of the keypad.)

QUICK TIP: To return quickly to the standard window setting [−10, 10, −10, 10], xscl = 1, yscl = 1, when either the Window screen or the Graph screen is displayed, press [F2] to access the ZOOM menu and then press 6 to select item 6, ZoomStd (Zoom Standard).

GRAPHING EQUATIONS

After entering an equation and setting a viewing window, you can view the graph of an equation.

Section 1.5, Example 5 Graph $y = 2x$ using a graphing calculator.

Equations are entered on the equation-editor screen. Press [◇] [Y =] to access this screen. If a plot is turned on, it should be turned off, or deselected, now. A check mark beside the name of a plot, such as Plot 1, indicates that it is currently selected. To deselect it, move the cursor to the plot's name on the equation-editor screen. Then press [F4]. There should now be no check mark beside the plot, indicating that it has been deselected. If there is currently an expression displayed for y1, clear it by positioning the cursor beside "y1 =" and pressing [CLEAR]. Do the same for expressions that appear on all other "y =" lines by using [▽] to move to a line and then pressing [CLEAR]. Then use [△] or [▽] to move the cursor beside "y1 =." Now enter y1 = 2x on the entry line of the equation-editor screen and paste it beside y1 = by pressing 2 [X] [ENTER].

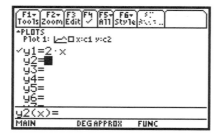

The standard $[-10, 10, -10, 10]$ window is a good choice for this graph. Either enter these dimensions in the WINDOW screen and then press $\boxed{\diamond}$ $\boxed{\text{GRAPH}}$ to see the graph or simply press $\boxed{\text{F2}}$ 6 to select the standard window and see the graph.

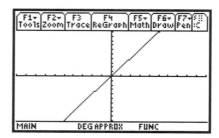

To edit an entry on the equation-editor screen, use $\boxed{\triangle}$ or $\boxed{\triangledown}$ to highlight it and then press $\boxed{\text{ENTER}}$. This copies the entry to the entry line where it can be edited as described on page 113 of this manual.

THE TABLE FEATURE

For an equation entered in the equation-editor screen, a table of x-and y-values can be displayed.

Section 1.5, Example 7 Create a table of ordered pairs that are solutions of the equation $y = -\dfrac{1}{2}x$. Use integer values of x beginning at -3.

First press $\boxed{\diamond}$ $\boxed{\text{Y} =}$ to access the equation-editor screen. Then clear any equations that are present. (See Example 5 above for the procedure to follow.) Next enter the equation by positioning the cursor beside "$y1 =$" and pressing $\boxed{(-)}$ 1 $\boxed{\div}$ 2 $\boxed{\text{X}}$.

Once the equation is entered, press $\boxed{\diamond}$ $\boxed{\text{TblSet}}$ to display the Table Setup screen. (TblSet is the green $\diamond$ operation associated with the $\boxed{\text{F4}}$ key.) The Table Setup screen can also be accessed by pressing $\boxed{\diamond}$ $\boxed{\text{TABLE}}$ $\boxed{\text{F2}}$. (TABLE is the green $\diamond$ operation associated with the $\boxed{\text{F5}}$ key.) You can choose to supply the x-values yourself or you can set the calculator to supply them.

If "Independent" is set to "Auto" on the Table Setup screen, the calculator will supply values for x, beginning with the value specified as tblStart and continuing by adding the value of Δtbl to the preceding value for x. For example, for the equation $y = -\dfrac{1}{2}x$ entered above, we will set the table to Auto mode and display a table of values that starts with $x = -3$ and adds 1 to the preceding x-value. If the table was previously set to Ask, the blinking cursor will be positioned over ASK on the Table Setup screen. Change this setting to AUTO by pressing $\boxed{\triangleright}$ 1 $\boxed{\text{ENTER}}$. Now the Table Setup screen must once again be accessed so that we can set tblStart and Δtbl. Enter a minimum x-value of -3, an increment of 1, and a Graph $< - >$ Table setting of OFF by first positioning the cursor beside tblStart and then pressing $\boxed{(-)}$ 3 $\boxed{\triangledown}$ 1 $\boxed{\triangledown}$ $\boxed{\triangleright}$ 1 $\boxed{\text{ENTER}}$.

Now press $\diamond$ $\boxed{\text{TABLE}}$ to view the table. You can use the $\boxed{\triangledown}$ and $\boxed{\triangle}$ keys to scroll through the table.

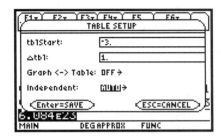

GRAPHS AS MODELS

A graphing calculator can plot data points and draw a line using those points.

Section 1.6, Example 7 *Weekly Newspapers.* The following table show the number of weekly newspapers in the United States for various years from 1960 to 2000. Use the data to draw a line graph.

Year	Number of Weekday Newspapers
1960	8174
1970	7612
1980	7954
1990	7606
2000	7689

We will enter the coordinates of the ordered pairs in the Data/Matrix editor. Press $\boxed{\text{APPS}}$ 6 3 to display the new data variable screen in the Data/Matrix editor. We must now enter a data variable name in the Variable box on this screen. The name can contain from 1 to 8 characters and cannot start with a numeral. Some names are preassigned to other uses on the TI-89. If you try to use one of these, you will get an error message. Press $\boxed{\triangledown}$ $\boxed{\triangledown}$ to move the cursor to the Variable box. We will name our data variable "news." To enter this name, first lock the alphabetic keys on by pressing $\boxed{\text{2nd}}$ $\boxed{\text{a-lock}}$. Then press $\boxed{\text{N}}$ $\boxed{\text{E}}$ $\boxed{\text{W}}$ $\boxed{\text{S}}$. Note that N, E, W, and S are the purple alphabetic operations associated with the 6, $\boxed{\div}$, $\boxed{\cdot}$, and 3 keys, respectively.

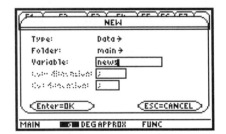

After typing the name of the data variable, unlock the alphabetic keys by pressing the purple $\boxed{\text{alpha}}$ key. Now press $\boxed{\text{ENTER}}$ $\boxed{\text{ENTER}}$ to go to the data-entry screen. Assuming the data variable name "news" has not previously been used in your calculator, this screen will contain empty data lists with row 1, column 1 highlighted. If entries have previously been made in a data variable named "news," they can be cleared by pressing $\boxed{\text{F1}}$ 8 $\boxed{\text{ENTER}}$.

We will enter the first coordinates (x-coordinates) of the points in column c1 and the second coordinates (y-coordinates) in c2. To enter the first x-coordinate, 1960, press 1 9 6 0 $\boxed{\text{ENTER}}$. Continue typing the x-values 1970, 1980, 1990, and 2000, each followed by $\boxed{\text{ENTER}}$. The entries can be followed by $\boxed{\triangledown}$ rather than $\boxed{\text{ENTER}}$ if desired. Press $\boxed{\triangleright}$ $\boxed{\triangle}$ $\boxed{\triangle}$ $\boxed{\triangle}$ $\boxed{\triangle}$ to move to the top of column c2. Type the y-values 8174, 7612, 7954, 7606, and 7689 in succession, each followed by $\boxed{\text{ENTER}}$ or $\boxed{\triangledown}$. Note that the coordinates of each point must be in the same position in both lists.

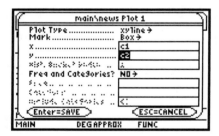

Next we access the Plot Setup screen by pressing $\boxed{\text{F2}}$. We will use Plot 1, which is highlighted. If any plot settings are currently entered beside "Plot 1,"" clear them by pressing $\boxed{\text{F3}}$. Clear settings shown beside any other plots as well by using $\boxed{\triangledown}$ to highlight each plot in turn and then pressing $\boxed{\text{F3}}$.

Now we define Plot 1. Use $\boxed{\triangle}$ to highlight Plot 1 if necessary. Then press $\boxed{\text{F1}}$ to display the Plot Definition screen. The item on the first line, Plot Type, is highlighted. We will choose a line graph, denoted xyline, by pressing $\boxed{\triangleright}$ 2. Now press $\boxed{\triangledown}$ to go to the next line, Mark. Here we select the type of mark or symbol that will be used to plot the points. We select a box by pressing $\boxed{\triangleright}$ 1. Now we must tell the calculator which columns of the data variable to use for the x- and y-coordinates of the points to be plotted. Press $\boxed{\triangledown}$ to move the cursor to the "x" line and enter c1 as the source of the x-coordinates by pressing $\boxed{\text{alpha}}$ C 1. (C is the purple alphabetic operation associated with the $\boxed{)}$ key.) Press $\boxed{\triangledown}$ $\boxed{\text{alpha}}$ C 2 to go the the "y" line and enter c2 as the source of the y-coordinates.

Save the plot definition and return to the Plot Setup screen by pressing $\boxed{\text{ENTER}}$ $\boxed{\text{ENTER}}$. Beside "Plot 1:" you will now see a shorthand notation for the definition of the plot.

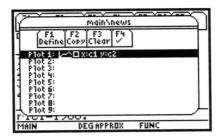

Now select a viewing window that will display all the data points. The years range from 1960 to 2000 and the numbers of newspapers range from 7606 to 8174, so one good choice is $[1950, 2010, 7500, 85000]$, xscl $= 10$, yscl $= 100$. Press $\boxed{\diamond}$ $\boxed{\text{GRAPH}}$ to see line graph of the data.

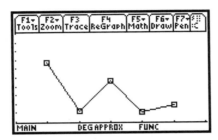

QUICK TIP: Instead of entering the window dimensions directly, we can press $\boxed{\text{F2}}$ 9 after entering the coordinates of the points in lists and defining Plot 1. This activates the ZoomData operation which automatically defines a viewing window that displays all the points and also displays the graph.

Turn off the plot as described on page 117 of this manual before graphing equations again.

THE TRACE FEATURE

The calculator's Trace feature displays the coordinates of the point indicated by the cursor.

Section 1.6, Example 8 *Model Rockets.* Suppose that a model rocket is launched upward with an initial velocity of 96 ft/sec. Its height in feet, h, after t seconds is given by

$$h = -16t^2 + 96t.$$

(a) For how long will the rocket climb?

(b) How high will the rocket go?

(c) After how long will the rocket reach the ground?

First we press $\boxed{\diamond}$ $\boxed{\text{Y} =}$ to go to the equation-editor screen. Enter y1 $= -16x^2 + 96x$ and graph the equation in the viewing window $[0, 10, 0, 200]$, yscl $= 10$. Note that the plots should be deselected. (See page 117 of this manual for the procedure.)

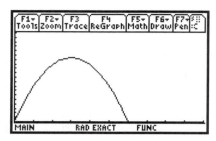

(a) The rocket climbs until the graph reaches the greatest y-value. The x-value associated with this y-value indicates how long the rocket climbs. To find this value, from the Graph screen press $\boxed{F3}$ to activate the Trace feature. The trace cursor appears on the graph. Use the right and left arrow keys to move the cursor to the highest point on the graph. The greatest y-value occurs when x is about 3, so we can say that the rocket climbs for about 3 seconds.

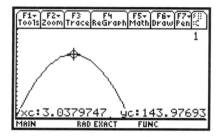

(b) To approximate how high the rocket will go, we read the greatest y-value in the Trace window above. Thus, we would say that the rocket will climb to a height of 144 feet.

(c) The rocket is on the ground when $y = 0$. The x-value associated with this y-value indicates how long it will take the rocket to reach the ground. We use Trace to find this x-value. From the Graph screen, press $\boxed{F3}$ and use the right arrow key to move the cursor to the point on the right side of the graph where y is approximately 0. We see that this y-value occurs when x is about 6, so we say that is will take about 6 seconds for the rocket to reach the ground.

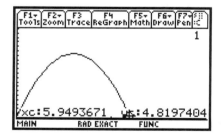

Chapter 2
Functions, Linear Equations, and Models

EVALUATING A FUNCTION

Function values can be found in several different ways on the TI-89.

Section 2.1, Example 6 For $f(a) = 2a^2 - 3a + 1$, find $f(3)$ and $f(-5.1)$.

One method for finding function values involves using function notation directly. To do this, first press $\boxed{\diamond}$ $\boxed{Y =}$ and clear any entries that are present. Also be sure the plots are deselected. (See page 117 of this manual for instructions for clearing equations and deselecting the plots.) Now enter the function on the equation-editor screen. Mentally replace a with x and $f(a)$ with y1. Then enter y1 $= 2x^2 - 3x + 1$. Now, to find $f(3)$, or y1(3), directly first press $\boxed{\text{HOME}}$ or $\boxed{\text{2nd}}$ $\boxed{\text{QUIT}}$ to go to the home screen. Then enter y1(3) on the entry line by pressing $\boxed{Y}$ 1 $\boxed{(}$ 3 $\boxed{)}$. Finally press $\boxed{\text{ENTER}}$. We see that y1(3)=10, or $f(3) = 10$.

To find $f(-5.1)$, or y1(-5.1), we can repeat the previous procedure using -5.1 in place of 3, or we can edit the previous entry. To edit, press $\boxed{\triangleright}$ to go to the right side of the previous entry on the entry line. Then press $\boxed{\triangleleft}$ $\boxed{\leftarrow}$ to delete the 3. Now press $\boxed{(-)}$ 5 $\boxed{.}$ 1 to replace 3 with -5.1. Finally press $\boxed{\text{ENTER}}$ to find that $y1(-5.1) = 68.32$, or $f(-5.1) = 68.32$.

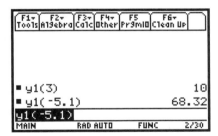

Another way to calculate a function value after the function has been entered on the equation-editor screen involves storing the input value in the calculator's memory. To find $f(3)$ for the function entered as y1 in this example, for instance, we can store 3 as the variable X by pressing 3 $\boxed{\text{STO} \triangleright}$ $\boxed{X}$ $\boxed{\text{ENTER}}$. Then find y1(x) when $x = 3$ by pressing $\boxed{Y}$ 1 $\boxed{(}$ $\boxed{X}$ $\boxed{)}$ $\boxed{\text{ENTER}}$.

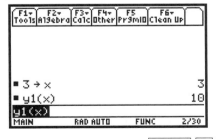

This computation can also be performed in a single step by pressing 3 $\boxed{\text{STO} \triangleright}$ $\boxed{X}$ $\boxed{\text{2nd}}$ $\boxed{:}$ $\boxed{Y}$ 1 $\boxed{(}$ $\boxed{X}$ $\boxed{)}$ $\boxed{\text{ENTER}}$. (The symbol : is the second operation associated with the 4 numeric key.)

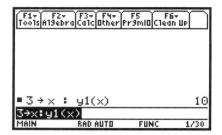

We can also find function values from the graph of the function.

Section 2.1, Example 7 Find $g(2)$ for $g(x) = 2x - 5$.

First press ◇ Y = to go to the equation editor screen and then clear any entries that are present. Also be sure that the plots are turned off. (See page 117 of this manual for instructions for clearing equations and turning off plots.) Now enter y1 = 2x − 5 and press F2 6 to graph this function in the standard viewing window. We will use the Value feature from the Math menu on the Graph screen to find the value of y1 when $x = 2$. This is $g(2)$. Press F5 1 to select Value. Press 2 ENTER. We now see xc:2, yc:−1 at the bottom of the screen. This indicates that when the x-coordinate on this graph is 2, the corresponding y-coordinate is −1, so $g(2) = -1$.

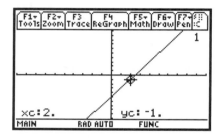

When using the Value feature, note that the x-value entered must be in the viewing window. That is, x must be a number between xmin and xmax.

SOLVING EQUATIONS GRAPHICALLY

We can use the Intersection feature from the Math menu on the Graph screen to solve equations.

Section 2.2, Example 3 Solve using a graphing calculator: $-\frac{3}{4}x + 6 = 2x - 1$.

On the equation-editor screen, clear any existing entries and then enter y1 $= -\frac{3}{4}x + 6$ and y2 = 2x − 1. Press F2 6 to graph these equations in the standard viewing window. The solution of the equation $-\frac{3}{4}x + 6 = 2x - 1$ is the first coordinate of the point of intersection of these graphs. To use the Intersection feature to find this point, first press F5 5 to select Intersection from the Math menu on the Graph screen. The query "1st curve?" appears at the bottom of the screen. The blinking cursor is positioned on the graph of y1. This is indicated by the 1 in the upper right-hand corner of the screen. Press ENTER to indicate that this is the first curve involved in the intersection. Next the query "2nd curve?" appears at the bottom of the screen. The blinking cursor is now positioned on the graph of y2 and the notation 2 should appear in the top right-hand corner of the screen. Press ENTER to indicate that this is the second curve. We identify the curves for the calculator since we could have more than two graphs on the screen at once. After we identify the second curve, the query "Lower bound?" appears at the bottom of the screen. Use the right and left arrow keys to move the blinking cursor to a point to the left of the point of intersection of the lines or type an x-value less than the x-coordinate of the point of intersection. Then press $\boxed{\text{ENTER}}$. Next the query "Upper bound?" appears. We give a lower and an upper bound since some pairs of curves have more than one point of intersection. Move the cursor to a point to the right of the point of intersection or type an x-value greater than the x-value of the point of intersection and press $\boxed{\text{ENTER}}$. Now the coordinates of the point of intersection appear at the bottom of the screen.

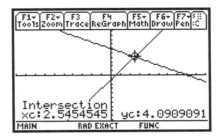

We see that $x = 2.5454545$, so the solution of the equation is 2.5454545.

We can check the solution by evaluating both sides of the equation $-\dfrac{3}{4}x + 6 = 2x - 1$ for this value of x. The first coordinate of the point of intersection has automatically been stored as xc in the calculator, so we evaluate y1 and y2 for this value of x. First press $\boxed{\text{HOME}}$ or $\boxed{\text{2nd}}$ $\boxed{\text{QUIT}}$ to go to the home screen. Then to evaluate y1 press $\boxed{\text{Y}}$ $\boxed{\text{1}}$ $\boxed{\text{(}}$ $\boxed{\text{X}}$ $\boxed{\text{alpha}}$ $\boxed{\text{C}}$ $\boxed{\text{)}}$ $\boxed{\text{ENTER}}$. To evaluate Y_2 press $\boxed{\text{Y}}$ $\boxed{\text{2}}$ $\boxed{\text{(}}$ $\boxed{\text{X}}$ $\boxed{\text{alpha}}$ $\boxed{\text{C}}$ $\boxed{\text{)}}$ $\boxed{\text{ENTER}}$. We see that y1 and y2 have the same value when $x = 2.5454545$, so the solution checks.

Note that although the procedure above verifies that 2.5454545 is the solution, it is actually an approximation of the solution. To find the exact solution we can solve the equation algebraically.

SOLVING FOR Y

The TI-89 graphs only functions, so an equation must be solved for the dependent variable before it can be entered into the calculator.

Section 2.3, Example 8 Graph $3x - 4y = 2y + 7$.

We must first use our formula-solving skills to solve this equation for y. We get $y = \dfrac{-3x + 7}{-6}$. Since $y = \dfrac{-3x + 7}{-6}$ is equivalent to $3x - 4y = 2y + 7$, the graphs of these equations will be the same. Thus, we can enter the equation y1 = $(-3x + 7)/-6$ on the equation-editor screen. We graph the equation in the standard viewing window.

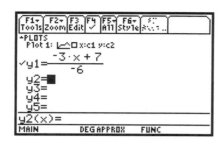
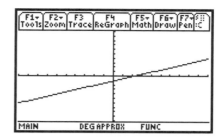

SQUARING THE VIEWING WINDOW

Section 2.5, Example 8 Determine whether the lines given by the equations $3x - y = 7$ and $x + 3y = 1$ are perpendicular, and check by graphing.

In the text each equation is solved for y in order to determine the slopes of the lines. We have $y = 3x - 7$ and $y = -\frac{1}{3}x + \frac{1}{3}$. Since $3\left(-\frac{1}{3}\right) = -1$, we know that the lines are perpendicular. To check this, we graph y1 $= 3x - 7$ and y2 $= -\frac{1}{3}x + \frac{1}{3}$. The graphs are shown on the right below in the standard viewing window.

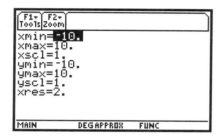
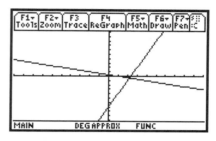

Note that the graphs do not appear to be perpendicular. This is due to the fact that, in the standard window, the distance between tick marks on the y-axis is about 1/2 the distance between tick marks on the x-axis. It is often desirable to choose window dimensions for which these distances are the same, creating a "square" window. On the TI-89 any window in which the ratio of the length of the y-axis to the length of the x-axis is 1/2 will produce this effect. This can be accomplished by selecting dimensions for which ymax $-$ ymin $= \frac{1}{2}$(xmax $-$ xmin). For example, the windows $[-12, 12, -6, 6]$ and $[-6, 6, -3, 3]$ are square.

When we change the window dimensions to $[-12, 12, -6, 6]$ and press $\boxed{\diamond}$ $\boxed{\text{GRAPH}}$, the graphs now appear to be perpendicular as shown on the right below. From the equation-editor, Window, or Graph screen, we could also press $\boxed{\text{F2}}$ 5 to select ZoomSqr. When this is done, the calculator will select a square window.

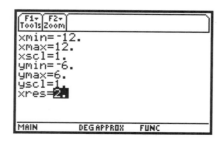
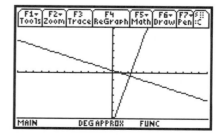

LINEAR REGRESSION

We can use the Linear Regression feature on the TI-89 to fit a linear equation to a set of data.

Section 2.6, Example 5 The amount of paper recovered in the United States for various years is shown in the following table.

Years	Amount of Paper Recovered (in millions of tons)
1988	26.2
1990	29.1
1992	34.0
1994	39.7
1996	43.1
1998	45.1
2000	49.4

(a) Fit a linear function to the data.

(b) Graph the function and use it to estimate the amount of paper that will be recovered in 2003.

(a) First press $\boxed{\diamond}$ $\boxed{Y =}$ to go to the equation-editor screen and clear any equations that are currently selected. A check mark to the left of an equation indicates that it is selected. (See page 117 of this manual for the procedure for clearing equations.) If you wish, instead of clearing an equation, you can deselect it. To do this, position the cursor beside the = sign and press $\boxed{F4}$. Note that there is no longer a check mark to the left of the equation, indicating that the equation has been deselected. The graph of an equation that has been deselected will not appear when $\boxed{\diamond}$ $\boxed{GRAPH}$ is pressed. A deselected equation can be selected again by positioning the cursor beside the = sign and pressing $\boxed{F4}$. Note that a check mark once again appears to the left of the equation.

Now press $\boxed{APPS}$ 6 3 to display a new data variable screen in the Data/Matrix editor and enter a data variable name. We will use "paper." Then go to the data-entry screen and enter the data in the table. (See pages 119 and 120 of this manual for the procedures for entering a data variable name and entering data.) We enter the number of years since 1988 in c1 and the number of millions of tons of paper recovered in c2.

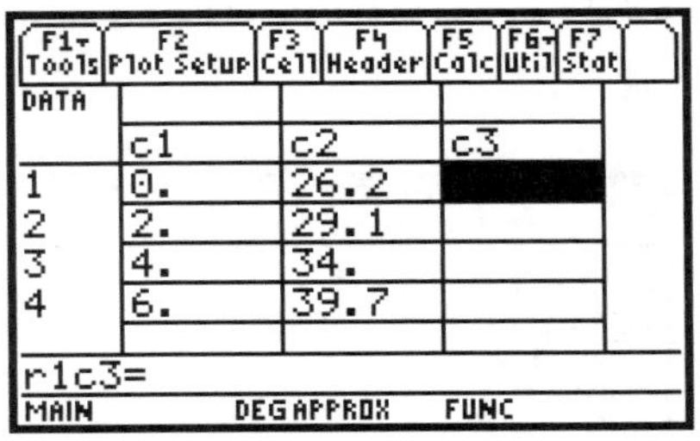

Now use the calculator's linear regression feature to fit a linear equation to the data. Press $\boxed{F5}$ to display the Calculate menu. Press $\boxed{\triangleright}$ 5 to select LinReg (linear regression). Then press $\boxed{\triangledown}$ $\boxed{\text{alpha}}$ $\boxed{C}$ 1 $\boxed{\triangledown}$ $\boxed{\text{alpha}}$ $\boxed{C}$ 2 to indicate that the data in c1 and c2 will be used for x and y, respectively. Press $\boxed{\triangledown}$ $\boxed{\triangleright}$ $\boxed{\triangledown}$ $\boxed{\text{ENTER}}$ to indicate that the regression equation should be copied to the equation-editor screen as y1. Finally press $\boxed{\text{ENTER}}$ again to see the STAT VARS screen which displays the coefficients a

and b of the regression equation $y = ax + b$. We see that the regression equation is $y = 1.976786x + 26.225$.

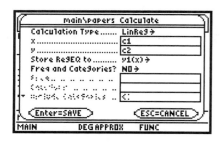 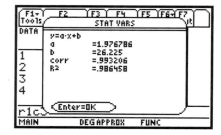

Note that values for "corr" (the correlation coefficient) and r^2 (the coefficient of determination) will also be displayed. These numbers indicate how well the regression line fits the data. While it is possible to suppress these numbers on some graphing calculators, this cannot be done on the TI-89.

(b) Now we will graph the regression equation. In order to see the data points along with the graph of the equation we will turn on and define a plot. To do this, from the STAT VARS screen first press ENTER F2 to go to the Plot Setup screen. We will define Plot 1, selecting scatter (a scatter diagram) for Type, a box for Mark, and c1 and c2 for x and y, respectively. (See page 120 of this manual for instructions.) Press ◊ WINDOW to go to the Window screen.

To select the dimensions of the viewing window notice that the years in the table range from 0 to 12 and the number of millions of tons of paper ranges from 26.2 to 49.4. We want to select dimensions that will include all of these values. One good choice is [0, 15, 0, 60], yscl = 10. Enter these dimensions in the Window screen. Then press ◊ GRAPH to see the graph of the regression line on the same axes as the data.

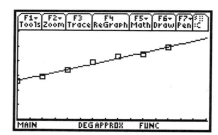

You can press ◊ Y =, if desired, to see the regression equation entered as y1 on the equation-editor screen.

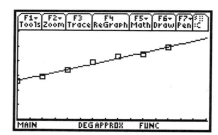

To estimate the amount of paper that will be recovered in 2003, evaluate the regression equation for $x = 15$. (2003 is 15 years after 1988.) Use any of the methods for evaluating a function presented earlier in this chapter. (See pages 123 and 124.) We will use the Value feature from the Math menu on the Graph screen. If you used ZoomData to select a window earlier, you might have to enter a new value for xmax so that $x = 15$ will be in the window.

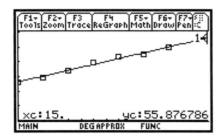

When $x = 15, y \approx 55.9$, so we estimate that there will be about 55.9 million tons of paper recovered in 2003.

Chapter 3
Systems of Equations and Problem Solving

SOLVING SYSTEMS OF EQUATIONS GRAPHICALLY

We can use the Intersection feature from the Math menu on the Graph screen of the TI-89 to solve a system of two equations in two variables.

Section 3.1, Example 4(a) Solve graphically:

$$y - x = 1,$$

$$y + x = 3.$$

We graph the equations in the same viewing window and then find the coordinates of the point of intersection. Remember that equations must be entered in "$y =$" form on the equation-editor screen, so we solve both equations for y. We have $y = x + 1$ and $y = -x + 3$. Enter these equations, graph them in the standard viewing window, and find their point of intersection as described on pages 124 and 125 of this manual. We see that the solution of the system of equations is $(1, 2)$.

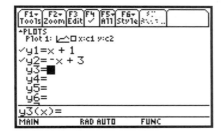   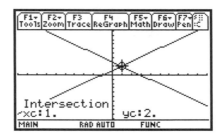

MODELS

Sometimes we model two situations with linear functions and then want to find the point of intersection of their graphs.

Section 3.1, Example 6 (d), (e) The numbers of U. S. travelers to Canada and to Europe are listed in the following table.

Year	U. S. Travelers to Canada (in millions)	U. S. Travelers to Europe (in millions)
1992	11.8	7.1
1994	12.5	8.2
1996	12.9	8.7
1998	14.9	11.1
2000	15.1	13.4

(d) Use linear regression to find two linear equations that can be used to estimate the number of U. S. travelers to Canada and Europe, in millions, x years after 1990.

(e) Use the equations found in part (d) to estimate the year in which the number of U. S. travelers to Europe will be the same as the number of U. S. travelers to Canada.

(d) Enter the data in the Data/Matrix editor as described on pages 119 and 120 of this manual. We will express the years as the number of years since 1990 (in other words, 1990 is year 0) and enter them in c1. Then enter the number of U. S. travelers to Canada, in millions, in c2 and the number of U. S. travelers to Europe,in millions, in c3.

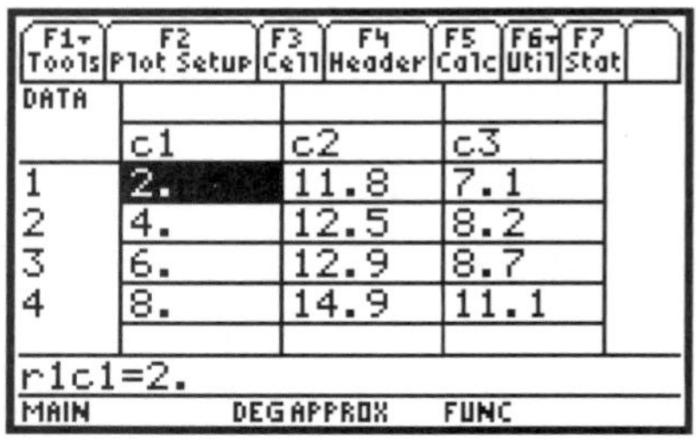

Now use linear regression to fit a linear function to the data in c1 and c2. The function should also be copied to the equation-editor screen. We will copy it as y1. See page 127 of this manual for the procedure to follow. We get y1 $= 0.45x + 10.74$.

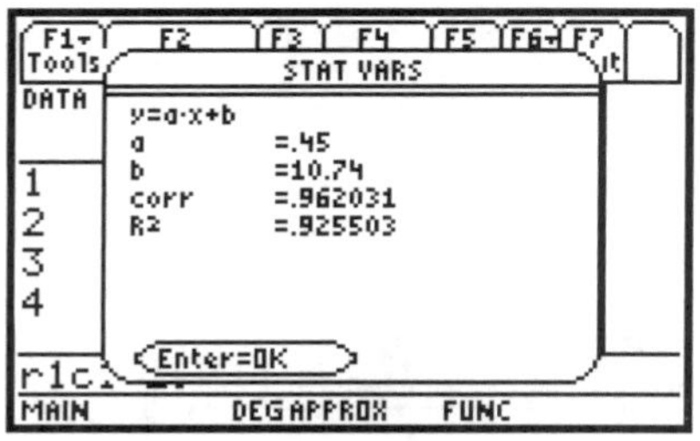

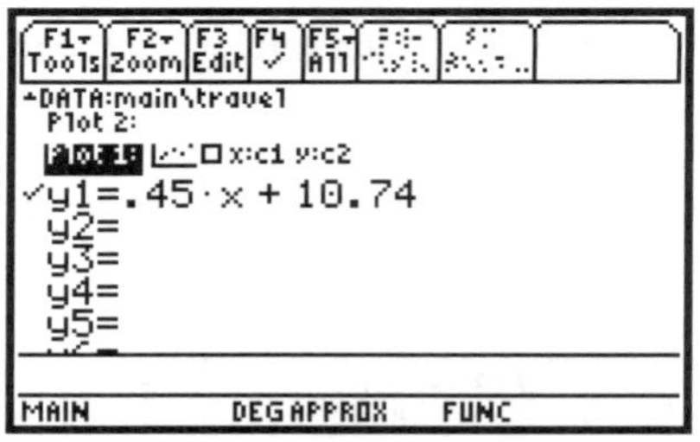

Next we fit a linear function to the data in c1 and c3, entering c1 as x and c3 as y on the Calculate screen. This function will be copied to the equation-editor screen as y2. To enter c3 as y, position the blinking cursor in the y box and press [alpha] [C] 3. To select y2 as the function to which the regression equation will be copied, position the cursor beside "Store Reg EQ to," press [▷], use the [▽] key to highlight y2(x) and press [ENTER]. We get y2 $= 0.775x + 5.05$.

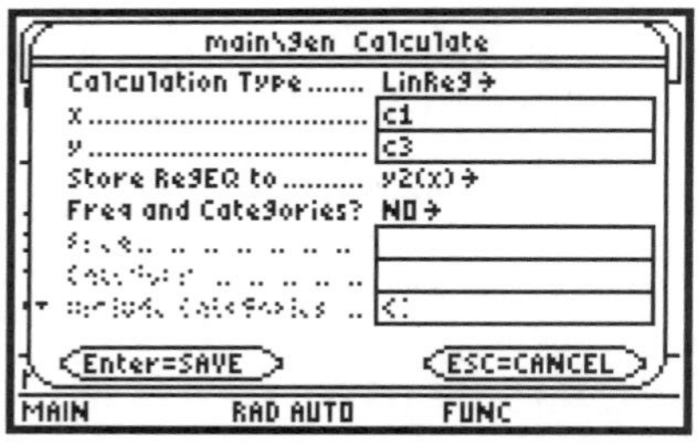

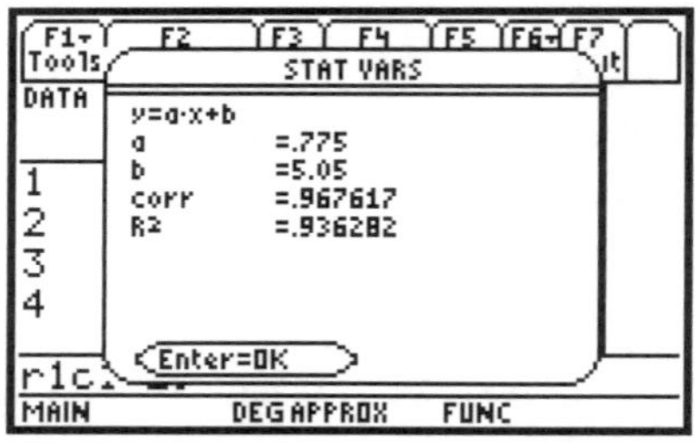

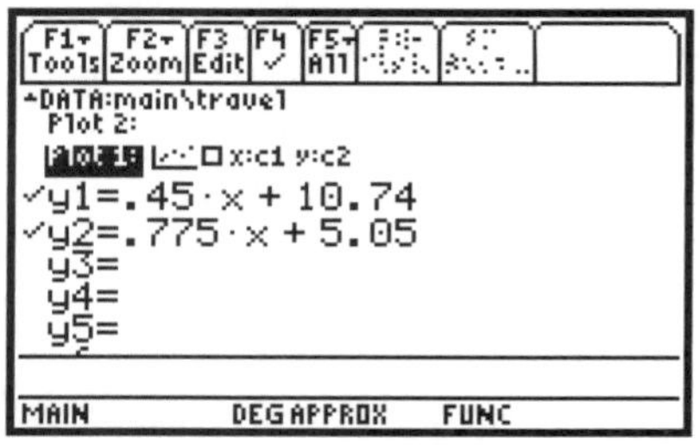

(e) To estimate the year in which the number of U. S. travelers to Europe will be the same as the number of U. S. travelers to Canada, we solve the system of equations

$$y = 0.45x + 10.74,$$
$$y = 0.775x + 5.05.$$

We graph the equations in the same viewing window and then use the Intersection feature to find their point of intersection. Through a trial-and-error process we find that $[0, 30, 0, 30]$, xscl $= 2$, yscl $= 2$, provides a good window in which to see this point. We see that the solution of the system of equations is approximately $(17.51, 18.62)$, so the number of U. S. travelers to Europe will be the same as the number of U. S. travelers to Canada about 17.5 years after 1990, or in 2008.

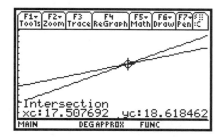

ELIMINATION USING MATRICES

Matrices with up to 999 rows and 99 columns can be entered on the TI-89. The row-equivalent operations necessary to write a matrix in row-echelon form or reduced row-echelon form can be performed on the calculator, or we can go directly to row-echelon form or reduced row-echelon form with a single command. We will illustrate the direct approach for finding reduced row-echelon form.

Section 3.6, Example 1 Solve the following system using a graphing calculator:

$$2x + 5y - 8z = 7,$$
$$3x + 4y - 3z = 8,$$
$$5y - 2x = 9.$$

First we rewrite the third equation in the form $ax + by + cz = d$:

$$2x + 5y - 8z = 7,$$
$$3x + 4y - 3z = 8,$$
$$-2x + 5y = 9.$$

Then we enter the coefficient matrix

$$\begin{bmatrix} 2 & 5 & -8 & 7 \\ 3 & 4 & -3 & 8 \\ -2 & 5 & 0 & 9 \end{bmatrix}$$

in the Data/Matrix editor. We will call the Matrix A. Press $\boxed{\text{APPS}}$ 6 3 $\boxed{\triangleright}$ 2 $\boxed{\triangledown}$ $\boxed{\triangledown}$ $\boxed{\text{alpha}}$ $\boxed{\text{A}}$ $\boxed{\triangledown}$ 3 $\boxed{\triangledown}$ 4 $\boxed{\text{ENTER}}$ $\boxed{\text{ENTER}}$ to go to the Data/Matrix editor and set up a matrix named A with 3 rows and 4 columns. If a matrix named A has previously been saved in your calculator, an error message will be displayed. If this happens, you can select a different name for the matrix we are about to enter or you can delete the current matrix A and then enter the new matrix as A. To delete a matrix press $\boxed{\text{2nd}}$ $\boxed{\text{VAR-LINK}}$, use $\boxed{\triangledown}$ to highlight the name of the matrix being deleted, and then press $\boxed{\text{F1}}$ 1 $\boxed{\text{ENTER}}$. (VAR-LINK is the second operation associated with the $\boxed{-}$ key.)

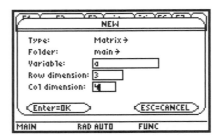

Enter the elements of the first row of the matrix by pressing 2 $\boxed{\text{ENTER}}$ 5 $\boxed{\text{ENTER}}$ $\boxed{(-)}$ 8 $\boxed{\text{ENTER}}$ 7 $\boxed{\text{ENTER}}$. The cursor moves to the element in the second row and first column of the matrix. Enter the elements of the second and third rows of the augmented matrix by typing each in turn followed by $\boxed{\text{ENTER}}$ as above. Note that the screen only displays three columns of the matrix. The arrow keys can be used to move the cursor to any element at any time.

Matrix operations are performed on the home screen and are found on the Math Matrix menu. Press $\boxed{\text{HOME}}$ or $\boxed{\text{2nd}}$ $\boxed{\text{QUIT}}$ to leave the matrix editor and go to this screen. Access the Math Matrix menu by pressing $\boxed{\text{2nd}}$ $\boxed{\text{MATH}}$ 4. (MATH is the second operation associated with the 5 numeric key.) The reduced row-echelon form command is item 4 on this menu. Copy it to the entry line of the home screen by pressing 4. We see the command "rref(" on the entry line.

Since we want to find reduced row-echelon form for matrix A, we enter A by pressing $\boxed{\text{alpha}}$ $\boxed{A}$ $\boxed{)}$. Finally press $\boxed{\text{ENTER}}$ to see reduced row echelon form of the original matrix. We see that the solution of the system of equations is $\left(\frac{1}{2}, 2, \frac{1}{2}\right)$ (or (0.5, 2, 0.5) if Auto or Approximate mode is selected rather than Exact mode).

Chapter 4
Inequalities and Problem Solving

GRAPHICAL SOLUTIONS OF INEQUALITIES

Solving inequalities graphically involves first finding a point of intersection.

Section 4.1, Example 4 Solve graphically: $16 - 7x \geq 10x - 4$.

Graph $y_1 = 16 - 7x$ and $y_2 = 10x - 4$ in the window $[-5, 5, -5, 15]$ and find the first coordinate of their point of intersection. It is approximately 1.1764706.

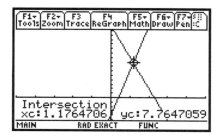

Observe that y_1 (on the graph that slants down from left to right) is greater than y_2 (on the graph that slants up from left to right) to the left of the point of intersection and $y_1 < y_2$ to the right of this point. Thus, the solution set will consist of all x-values to the left of 1.1764706 and also the value 1.1764706 itself since the inequality symbol is $\geq$, or $(-\infty, 1.1764706]$.

INEQUALITIES IN TWO VARIABLES

The solution set of an inequality in two variables can be graphed on the TI-89.

Section 4.4, Example 4 Use a graphing calculator to graph the inequality $8x + 3y > 24$.

First we write the related equation, $8x + 3y = 24$, and solve it for y. We get $y = -\dfrac{8}{3}x + 8$. We will enter this as $y1$. Press $\boxed{\diamond}$ $\boxed{Y =}$ to go to the equation-editor screen. If there is currently an entry for $y1$, clear it. Also clear or deselect any other equations that are entered. Now enter $y_1 = -\dfrac{8}{3}x + 8$. Since the inequality states that $8x + 3y > 24$, or y is *greater than* $-\dfrac{8}{3}x + 8$, we want to shade the half-plane above the graph of $y1$. To do this, use the cursor to highlight $y1$. Then press $\boxed{2\text{nd}}$ $\boxed{\text{F6}}$ to display the Style menu. Choose item 7, Above, by pressing 7. (To shade below a line we would press 8 to select Below.) Then press $\boxed{\text{F2}}$ 6 to see the graph of the inequality in the standard viewing window.

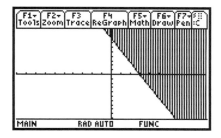

Note that when the "shade above" Style is selected it is not also possible to select the "Dot" style so we must keep in mind the fact that the line $y = -\dfrac{8}{3}x + 8$ is not included in the graph of the inequality. If you graphed this inequality by hand, you would draw a dashed line.

SYSTEMS OF LINEAR INEQUALITIES

We can graph systems of inequalities by shading the solution set of each inequality in the system with a different pattern. When the "shade above" or "shade below" style options are selected the calculator rotates through four shading patterns. Vertical lines shade the first function, horizontal lines the second, negatively sloping diagonal lines the third, and positively sloping diagonal lines the fourth. These patterns repeat if more than four functions are graphed.

Section 4.4, Example 8 Graph the system
$$x + y \le 4,$$
$$x - y < 4.$$

First graph the equation $x + y = 4$, entering it in the form $y = -x + 4$. We determine that the solution set of $x + y \le 4$ consists of all points on or below the line $x + y = 4$, or $y = -x + 4$, so we select the "shade below" style for this function. Next graph $x - y = 4$, entering it in the form $y = x - 4$. The solution set of $x - y < 4$ is all points above the line $x - y = 4$, or $y = x - 4$, so for this function we choose the "shade above" style. (See Example 4 above for instructions on selecting styles.) Now press $\boxed{\text{F2}}$ 6 to display the solution sets of each inequality in the system and the region where they overlap in the standard viewing window. The region of overlap is the solution set of the system of inequalities. Keep in mine that the line $x + y = 4$, or $y = -x + 4$, is part of the solution set while $x - y = 4$, or $y = x - 4$, is not.

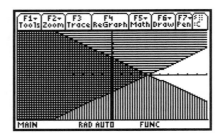

Chapter 5
Polynomials and Polynomial Functions

EVALUATING A POLYNOMIAL FUNCTION

We can use a table set in Ask mode to evaluate a polynomial function.

Section 5.1, Example 4 Find $P(-5)$ for the polynomial function given by $P(x) = -x^2 + 4x - 1$.

To use a table to find this function value, first enter $y1 = -x^2 + 4x - 1$ on the equation-editor screen. Then press $\boxed{\diamond}$ $\boxed{\text{TblSet}}$ to display the table set-up screen. To set up a table in which you choose the x-values that are entered, set Independent to Ask by positioning the cursor beside Independent and pressing $\boxed{\triangleright}$ 2 $\boxed{\text{ENTER}}$. In Ask mode the calculator disregards the setting of tblStart and Δtbl.

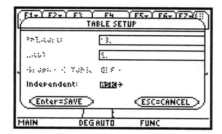

Now press $\boxed{\diamond}$ $\boxed{\text{TABLE}}$ to view the table. If you select Ask before a table is displayed for the first time on your calculator, a blank table is displayed. If a table has previously been displayed, the table you now see will continue to show the values in the previous table.

Values for x can be entered in the x-column of the table and the corresponding values for $y1$ will be displayed in the $y1$-column. To enter -5, for instance, press $\boxed{(-)}$ 5 $\boxed{\text{ENTER}}$. We see that $P(-5) = -46$. Any additional x-values that are displayed are from a table that was previously displayed on the Auto setting.

CHECKING OPERATIONS ON POLYNOMIALS

A graphing calculator can be used to check operations on polynomials.

Section 5.1, Example 9 Add: $(-3x^3 + 2x - 4) + (4x^3 + 3x^2 + 2)$.

This addition is carried out in the text, and the result is $x^3 + 3x^2 + 2x - 2$. There are several ways in which we can use a graphing calculator to check this result. One of these is to compare the graphs of $y1 = (-3x^3 + 2x - 4) + (4x^3 + 3x^2 + 2)$ and $y2 = x^3 + 3x^2 + 2x - 2$. This is most easily done when different graph styles are used for the graphs.

Eight graph styles can be selected on the TI-89. The **path graph style** can be used, along with the line style, to determine whether graphs coincide. First, on the equation-editor screen, enter $y1 = (-3x^3 + 2x - 4) + (4x^3 + 3x^2 + 2)$ and $y2 = x^3 + 3x^2 + 2x - 2$. We will select the path style from the style menu for $y2$. To do this, highlight the expression for $y2$ and then press $\boxed{\text{2nd}}$ $\boxed{\text{F6}}$ 6 $\boxed{\text{ENTER}}$ or press $\boxed{\text{2nd}}$ $\boxed{\text{F6}}$ $\boxed{\triangledown}$ $\boxed{\triangledown}$ $\boxed{\triangledown}$ $\boxed{\triangledown}$ $\boxed{\triangledown}$ $\boxed{\text{ENTER}}$.

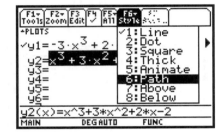

The calculator will graph $y1$ first as a solid line. Then $y2$ will be graphed as the circular cursor traces the leading edge of the graph, allowing us to determine visually whether the graphs coincide. In this case, the graphs appear to coincide, so the factorization is probably correct.

We can also check the addition by **subtracting** the result from the original sum. With $y1$ and $y2$ entered as described above, position the cursor beside "$y3 =$" and enter $y_3 = y1 - y2$ by pressing $\boxed{\text{Y}}$ 1 $\boxed{-}$ $\boxed{\text{Y}}$ 2 $\boxed{\text{ENTER}}$. If the subtraction is correct, $y1 = y2$, so $y3 = 0$ and the graph of $y3$ will be $y = 0$, or the x-axis. Since we are interested only in values of $y3$, deselect $y1$ and $y2$ as described on page 127 of this manual. Select the path graph style for $y3$ as described above.

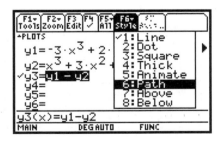

Now press $\boxed{\diamond}$ $\boxed{\text{GRAPH}}$ and determine if the graph of $y3$ is traced over the x-axis. Since it is, the sum is correct.

We can also use a table of values to **compare values** of $y1$ and $y2$. If the expressions for $y1$ and $y2$ are the same for each given x-value, the result checks. If you deselected $y1$ and $y2$ to check the sum using subtraction as described above, select them again now. Then look at a table set in Auto mode. Since the values of $y1$ and $y2$ are the same for each given x-value, the result checks.

Scrolling through the table to look at additional values makes this conclusion more certain.

x	y1	y2	
-3.	-8.	-8.	
-2.	-2.	-2.	
-1.	-2.	-2.	
0.	-2.	-2.	
1.	4.	4.	

x= -3.

MAIN   DEG AUTO   FUNC

We can also check the sum in Example 9 using a **horizontal split screen**, or **top-bottom split screen**. We will choose to display the graph in the top half of the screen and a table of values in the bottom half.

First enter $y1$ and $y2$ as described above. Then set up a table in Auto mode. (See page 118.) We will use tblStart $= -3$ and Δtbl $= 1$. To select the top-bottom split-screen option, first press $\boxed{\text{MODE}}$ $\boxed{\text{F2}}$ to access the second page of the Mode screen. Then press $\boxed{\triangleright}$ 2 to select a screen split into a top and a bottom portion. Next press $\boxed{\triangledown}$ $\boxed{\triangleright}$ 4 $\boxed{\triangledown}$ $\boxed{\triangleright}$ 5 $\boxed{\text{ENTER}}$ to select the graph to be displayed in the top portion of the screen and a table of values in the bottom portion. It might be necessary to press $\boxed{\diamond}$ $\boxed{\text{TABLE}}$ to see the table. We show the functions graphed in the standard window.

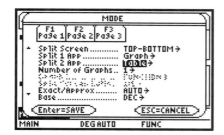 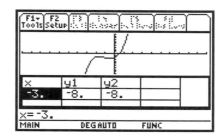

We can also use a **vertical split screen**, of **left-right split screen** to check Example 9. First enter $y1$, $y2$, and $y3$ as described above and deselect $y1$ and $y2$. Then press $\boxed{\text{MODE}}$ $\boxed{\text{F2}}$ to display the second Mode screen. Press $\boxed{\triangleright}$ to select left-right. Then select Graph for Split 1 App and Table for Split 2 App. Now press $\boxed{\text{ENTER}}$ to see the graph of $y3$ on the left side of the screen and a table of values for $y3$ on the right side. As we did above, we use show the graph in the standard window and use a table set in Auto mode with tblStart $= -3$ and Δtbl $= 1$. Since the graph appears to be $y = 0$, or the x-axis, and all of the $y3$-values in the table are 0, we confirm that the result is correct.

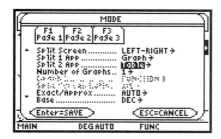

In order to return to a full screen, return to the second Mode screen and select Full for the Split Screen option.

FINDING THE ZEROS OF A FUNCTION

We can use the Zero feature from the Math menu on the Graph screen to find the zeros of a function.

Section 5.3, Example 2 Find the zeros of the function given by $f(x) = x^3 - 3x^2 - 4x + 12$.

First we graph the function in a viewing window that shows the x-intercepts clearly. Through a trail-and-error process we find that $[-5, 5, -20, 20]$, yscl $= 10$, is a good choice. We see that the function has three zeros. They appear to be about -2, 2, and 3.

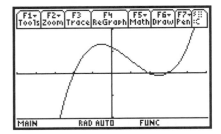

We will find the zero near -2 first. Press [F5] 2 to select the Zero feature from the Math menu. We are prompted to select a lower bound. This means that we must choose an x-value that is to the left of -2 on the x-axis. This can be done by using the left- and right-arrow keys to move to a point on the curve to the left of -2 or by keying in a value less than -2.

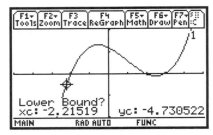

Once this is done press [ENTER]. Now we are prompted to select an upper bound that is to the right of -2 on the x-axis. Again, this can be done by using the arrow keys to move to a point on the curve to the right of -2 or by keying in a value greater that -2.

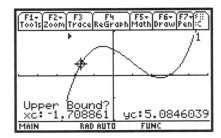

Press [ENTER] again. We see that $y = 0$ when $x = -2$, so -2 is a zero of the function f.

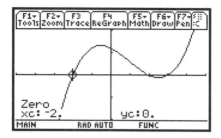

Select Zero from the Math menu a second time to find the zero near 2 and a third time to find the zero near 3. We see that the other two zeros are exactly 2 and 3.

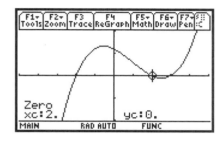
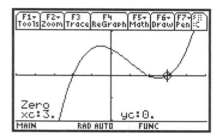

POLYNOMIAL REGRESSION

The TI-89 has the capability to use regression to fit nonlinear polynomial equations to data.

Section 5.8, Example 4(a) The number of bachelor's degrees earned in the biological and life sciences for various years is shown in the following table. Fit a polynomial function of degree 3 (cubic) to the data.

Year	Number of Bachelor's Degrees Earned in Biological/Life Science
1971	35,743
1976	54,275
1980	46,370
1986	38,524
1990	37,204
1994	51,383
2000	63,532

First enter the data in the Data/Matrix editor with the number of years since 1970 in c1 and the number of degree earned, in thousands, in c2. (See pages 119 and 120 of this manual.) A polynomial in one variable of degree 3 is called a cubic, so we will select cubic regression, denoted CubicReg, from the Calculate menu. This is item 3 under CalculationType. The calculator returns the coefficients for a cubic function of the form $f(x) = ax^3 + bx^2 + cx + d$. Rounding the coefficients to the nearest thousandth, we have $f(x) = 0.009x^3 - 0.371x^2 + 4.176x + 34.415$. We can see the coefficients given to more decimal places on the equation-editor screen, if desired.

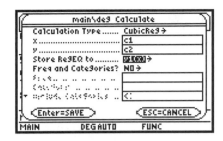 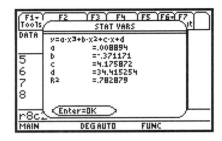

We can use methods discussed earlier in this manual to estimate and predict function values and to find the year or years in which a specific function value occurs.

Chapter 6
Rational Equations and Functions

GRAPHING IN DOT MODE

Consider the graph of the function $T(t) = \dfrac{t^2 + 5t}{2t + 5}$ in Section 6.1, Example 1. Enter $y = (x^2 + 5x)/(2x + 5)$ and graph it in the window $[-5, 5, -5, 5]$.

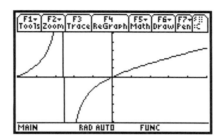

Note that a vertical line that is not part of the graph appears on the screen along with the two branches of the graph. The reason for this is discussed in the text.

This line will not appear if we change from Line style to Dot style. After entering $y1 = (x^2 + 5x)/(2x + 5)$, highlight $y1$ on the equation-editor screen. Then access the Style menu by pressing $\boxed{\text{2nd}}$ $\boxed{\text{F6}}$. Press 2 to select Dot style. Now press $\boxed{\diamond}$ $\boxed{\text{GRAPH}}$ to see the graph of the function in Dot style.

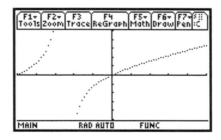

Chapter 7
Exponents and Radical Functions

RADICAL EXPRESSIONS AND RATIONAL EXPONENTS

On the TI-89 we can enter an expression containing a square root using radical notation or rational exponents. For example, we can enter $y = \sqrt{x-3}$ using radical notation or as $y = (x-2)^{1/2}$ or as $y = (x-3)^{.5}$. To enter $= \sqrt{x-3}$, press $\boxed{\text{2nd}}$ $\boxed{\sqrt{}}$ $\boxed{\text{X}}$ $\boxed{-}$ $\boxed{3}$ $\boxed{)}$. ($\sqrt{}$ is the second operation associated with the $\boxed{\times}$ multiplication key.) Note that the calculator supplies the left parenthesis along with the radical symbol and we add a right parenthesis after entering the radicand. To enter $y = (x-3)^{1/2}$, press $\boxed{(}$ $\boxed{\text{X}}$ $\boxed{-}$ $\boxed{3}$ $\boxed{)}$ $\boxed{\wedge}$ $\boxed{(}$ $\boxed{1}$ $\boxed{\div}$ $\boxed{2}$ $\boxed{)}$. Note that both the radicand and the rational exponent are enclosed in parentheses. To enter $y = (x-3)^{.5}$, press $\boxed{(}$ $\boxed{\text{X}}$ $\boxed{-}$ $\boxed{3}$ $\boxed{)}$ $\boxed{\wedge}$ $\boxed{\cdot}$ 5. When the exponent is in decimal notation it is not necessary to enclose it in parentheses.

We use a rational exponent to enter a cube root as well as any other higher order roots. For example, to enter $y = \sqrt[3]{x+5}$ we enter $y = (x+5)^{1/3}$ by pressing $\boxed{(}$ $\boxed{\text{X}}$ $\boxed{+}$ $\boxed{5}$ $\boxed{)}$ $\boxed{\wedge}$ $\boxed{(}$ $\boxed{1}$ $\boxed{\div}$ $\boxed{3}$ $\boxed{)}$. Since we cannot enter exact decimal notation for $1/3$, we cannot use decimal notation for the exponent in this case.

We can enter $f(x) = \sqrt[4]{2x-7}$, as in Section 7.2, Example 3, as $f(x) = (2x-7)^{1/4}$ or as $f(x) = (2x-7)^{.25}$.

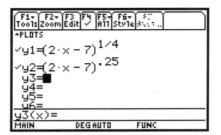

Chapter 8
Quadratic Functions and Equations

FINDING THE VERTEX

We can use a graphing calculator to find the vertex of a quadratic function. We do this by using the Maximum or Minimum feature from the Math menu or the Graph screen.

Section 8.7, Example 4 Use a graphing calculator to determine the vertex of the graph of the function given by $f(x) = -2x^2 + 10x - 7$.

The coefficient of x^2 is negative, so we know that the graph of the function opens down and, thus, has a maximum value. Clear or deselect any functions previously entered on the equation-editor screen. Then enter $y = -2x^2 + 10x - 7$. Choose a viewing window that shows the vertex. One good choice is $[-3, 7, -10, 10]$.

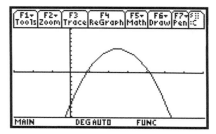

Now select the Maximum feature from the CALC menu by pressing $\boxed{\text{F5}}$ 4. We are prompted to select a lower bound for the vertex. Use the arrow keys to move the cursor to a point on the parabola to the left of the vertex or key in an x-value that is less than the x-coordinate of the vertex.

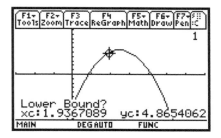

Press $\boxed{\text{ENTER}}$. Next we are prompted to select an upper bound. Move the cursor to a point on the parabola to the right of the vertex or key in an x-value that is greater than the x-coordinate of the vertex.

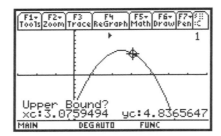

Press ENTER. We see that the maximum function value is 5.5, and it occurs when x is 2.5. Thus, the vertex of the graph of $f(x) = -2x^2 + 10x - 7$ is $(2.5, 5.5)$.

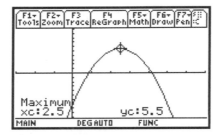

Minimum function values are found in a similar manner. Select the Minimum feature from the Math menu on the Graph screen by pressing F5 3.

QUADRATIC REGRESSION

Regression can be used to fit a quadratic function to data when three or more data points are given.

Section 8.8, Example 4(c) According to the Centers for Disease Control and Prevention, the percent of high school students who reported having smoked a cigarette in the preceding 30 days declined from 1997 to 2001, after rising in the first part of the 1990s. Use the REGRESSION feature of a graphing calculator to fit a quadratic function $H(x)$ to all the given data in the following table.

Years after 1991	Percent of High School Students Who Smoked a Cigarette in the Preceding 30 Days
0	27.5
2	30.5
4	34.9
6	36.4
8	34.9
10	28.5

We enter the data in the Data/Matrix editor as described on pages 119 and 120 of this manual.

Then select QuadReg as the CalculationType from the Calc menu by pressing [F5] [▷] 9. Specify the sources of x and y and a function name to which the equation will be stored. (See page 127 of this manual for the procedure.) Then press [ENTER] [ENTER]. The calculator returns the coefficients of a quadratic function $y = ax^2 + bx + c$. We have $H(x) = -0.315179x^2 + 3.433214x + 26.507143$.

The function can be evaluated using one of the methods on pages 123, 124, and 137.

Chapter 9
Exponential and Logarithmic Functions

COMPOSITE FUNCTIONS

For functions y_1 and y_2, when we enter $y_1(y_2)$ on a calculator we are entering the composition $y_1 \circ y_2$. The composite functions found in Section 9.1, Example 2 are checked using tables on a graphing calculator. To check that $f \circ g = \sqrt{x-1}$ when $f(x) = \sqrt{x}$ and $g(x) = x - 1$, enter $y_1 = \sqrt{x}$, $y_2 = x - 1$, $y_3 = \sqrt{x-1}$, and $y_4 = y_1(y_2)$ on the equation-editor screen. To enter y_4, position the cursor beside $y4 =$, clear any existing entry, and press $\boxed{Y}\,1\,\boxed{(}\,\boxed{Y}\,2\,\boxed{(}\,\boxed{X}\,\boxed{)}\,\boxed{)}\,\boxed{ENTER}$. Then compare the values of y_3 and y_4 in a table. We show a table with tblStart $= 1$, Δtbl $= 0.5$, and Independent set on Auto. Use the $\boxed{\triangleright}$ key to scroll across the table to see the $y3$- and $y4$-columns.

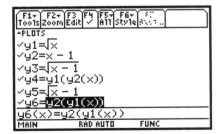

Similarly, to check that $g \circ f(x) = \sqrt{x} - 1$, also enter $y_5 = \sqrt{x} - 1$ and $y_6 = y_2(y_1)$. To enter y_6, position the cursor beside $y6 =$, clear any existing entry, and press $\boxed{Y}\,2\,\boxed{(}\,\boxed{Y}\,1\,\boxed{(}\,\boxed{X}\,\boxed{)}\,\boxed{)}\,\boxed{ENTER}$.

GRAPHING FUNCTIONS AND THEIR INVERSES

We can graph the inverse of a function using the DrawInv feature from the Draw menu on the Graph screen.

Section 9.1, Example 9(c) Graph the inverse of the function $g(x) = x^3 + 2$.

We will graph $g(x)$, $g^{-1}(x)$, and the line $y = x$ on the same screen. Press $\boxed{\diamond}\,\boxed{Y=}$ to go to the equation-editor screen and clear or deselect any existing entries. Then enter $y_1 = x^3 + 2$ and $y_2 = x$. Select a square window by pressing $\boxed{F2}$ 5. Now paste the DrawInv command from the Draw menu to the home screen by pressing $\boxed{2nd}\,\boxed{F6}$ 3. Indicate that we want to draw the inverse of y_1 by pressing $\boxed{\text{Y}}$ $\boxed{1}$ $\boxed{(}$ $\boxed{\text{X}}$ $\boxed{)}$. Finally press $\boxed{\text{ENTER}}$ to see the graph of y_1^{-1} along with the graphs of y_1 and y_2. We show a window that has been squared from the standard window.

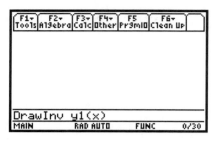 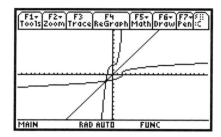

The drawing of y_1^{-1} can be cleared from the Graph screen by pressing $\boxed{\text{F4}}$ (ReGraph) or by pressing $\boxed{\text{2nd}}$ $\boxed{\text{F6}}$ to display the Draw menu and then pressing 1 to select ClrDraw. The ClrDraw command can also be accessed from the Catalog. From the home screen, press $\boxed{\text{CATALOG}}$ $\boxed{\text{C}}$, scroll to ClrDraw, and press $\boxed{\text{ENTER}}$ $\boxed{\text{ENTER}}$.

GRAPHING LOGARITHMIC FUNCTIONS

Section 9.3, Example 4 Graph: $f(x) = \log \dfrac{x}{5} + 1$.

We enter $y = \log(x/5) + 1$ on the equation-editor screen by positioning the cursor beside one of the function names and pressing $\boxed{\text{2nd}}$ $\boxed{\text{a-lock}}$ $\boxed{\text{L}}$ $\boxed{\text{O}}$ $\boxed{\text{G}}$ $\boxed{(}$ $\boxed{\text{X}}$ $\boxed{\div}$ $\boxed{5}$ $\boxed{)}$ $\boxed{+}$ $\boxed{1}$ $\boxed{\text{ENTER}}$. Note that $x/5$ must be enclosed in parentheses as shown. If parentheses are not used, the function entered will be $y = \dfrac{\log x}{5} + 1$. Clear or deselect any other functions. We show the function graphed in the window $[-2, 10, -5, 5]$.

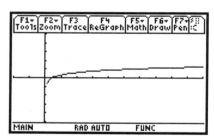

MORE ON GRAPHING

Section 9.5, Example 4 Graph: $f(x) = e^{-0.5x} + 1$.

We enter $y = e^{-0.5x}$ on the equation-editor screen by positioning the cursor beside one of the function names and pressing $\boxed{\diamond}$ $\boxed{e^x}$ $\boxed{(-)}$ $\boxed{.}$ 5 $\boxed{\text{X}}$ $\boxed{)}$ $\boxed{+}$ 1 $\boxed{\text{ENTER}}$. (Clear or deselect any other functions.) Select a window and press $\boxed{\text{GRAPH}}$. We show the function graphed in the window $[-5, 5, -2, 10]$.

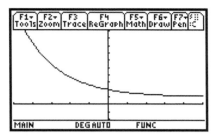

Section 9.5, Example 5(b) Graph: $f(x) = \ln(x + 3)$.

We enter $y = \ln(x + 3)$ on the equation-editor screen by positioning the cursor beside one of the function names and pressing

[2nd] [LN] [X] [+] [3] [)] [ENTER]. (Clear or deselect any other functions.) Select a window and press [◇] [GRAPH]. We show

the function graphed in the window $[-5, 10, -5, 5]$.

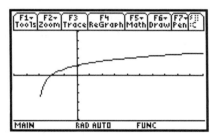

Section 9.5, Example 6 Graph: $f(x) = \log_7 x + 2$.

To use a graphing calculator we must first change the logarithmic base to e or 10. We will use e here. Recall that the change of

base formula is $\log_b M = \dfrac{\log_a M}{\log_a b}$, where a and b are any logarithmic bases and M is any positive number. Let $a = e$, $b = 7$, and

$M = x$ and substitute in the change-of-base formula. After clearing or deselecting previously entered functions, enter $y_1 = \dfrac{\ln x}{\ln 7} + 2$

on the equation-editor screen by positioning the cursor beside $y_1 =$ and pressing [2nd] [LN] [X] [)] [÷] [2nd] [LN] [7] [)] [+] [2]

[ENTER]. Note that the parentheses must be closed in both the numerator and the denominator. Select a viewing window and

press [◇] [GRAPH]. We show the graph in the window $[-2, 8, -2, 5]$.

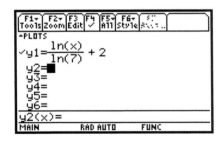
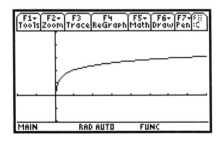

EXPONENTIAL REGRESSION

The TI-89 has an exponential regression feature.

Section 9.7, Example 9(a) In 1800, over 500,000 Tule elk inhabited the state of California. By the late 1800s, after the California Gold Rush, there were fewer than 50 elk remaining in the state. In 1978, wildlife biologists introduced a herd of 10 Tule elk into the Point Reyes National Seashore near San Francisco. By 1982, the herd had grown to 24 elk. There were 70 elk in 1986, 200 in 1996, and 500 in 2002. Use regression to fit an exponential function to the data and graph the function.

We enter the data as described on pages 119 and 120 of this manual. Let x represent the number of years since 1978.

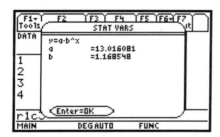

Now press F5 to go to the Calculate screen. Select ExpReg from the CalculationType menu by pressing ▷ 4. Enter the sources of x and y and the function name to which the equation will be saved. Then press ENTER . The calculator returns the values of a and b for the exponential function $y = ab^x$. We have $y = 13.016081(1.168548)^x$. We graph the equation in the window $[-2, 40, -5, 1000]$, xscl $= 5$, yscl $= 100$.

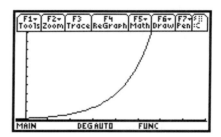

This function can be evaluated using one of the methods on pages 123, 124, and 137.

Chapter 10
Sequences, Series, and the Binomial Theorem

SEQUENCE MODE

To enter a sequence in a graphing calculator, first select Seq (Sequence) mode for the Graph setting. Press $\boxed{\text{MODE}}$ $\boxed{\triangleright}$ 4 $\boxed{\text{ENTER}}$.

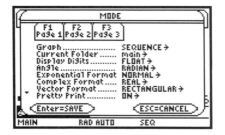

The function names that appear on the equation-editor screen when $\boxed{\diamond}$ $\boxed{\text{Y} =}$ is pressed are $u1$, $u2$, and so on rather than y_1, y_2, and so on. In addition we will use the variable n instead of x.

Section 10.1, Example 1 Find the first four terms and the 13th term of the sequence for which the general term is given by $a_n = (-1)^n n^2$.

After selecting Sequence mode, press $\boxed{\diamond}$ $\boxed{\text{Y} =}$ to go to the sequence-editor screen, enter the general term of the sequence beside "$u1 =$" by pressing $\boxed{(}$ $\boxed{(-)}$ 1 $\boxed{)}$ $\boxed{\wedge}$ $\boxed{\text{alpha}}$ $\boxed{\text{N}}$ $\boxed{\times}$ $\boxed{\text{alpha}}$ $\boxed{\text{N}}$ $\boxed{\wedge}$ 2 $\boxed{\text{ENTER}}$.

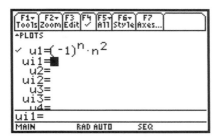

Now set up a table with Independent set to Ask. (See page 118 of this manual.) To see the first four terms and the 13th term of the sequence enter 1, 2, 3, 4, and 13 for n in the table.

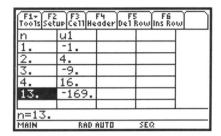

THE SEQUENCE FEATURE

The Sequence feature of the TI-89 writes the terms of a sequence as a list. This feature can be used even if the calculator is not in Sequence mode.

Section 10.1, Example 2 Use a graphing calculator to find the first five terms of the sequence for which the general term is given by $a_n = n/(n+1)^2$.

From the home screen we will access the Sequence feature from the Math List menu and copy it to the entry line by pressing $\boxed{\text{2nd}}$ $\boxed{\text{Math}}$ 3 1. Now enter the general term of the sequence, the variable, and the values of the variable for the first and last terms we wish to calculate, all separated by commas. Press $\boxed{\text{alpha}}$ $\boxed{\text{N}}$ $\boxed{\div}$ $\boxed{(}$ $\boxed{\text{alpha}}$ $\boxed{\text{N}}$ $\boxed{+}$ 1 $\boxed{)}$ $\boxed{\wedge}$ 2 $\boxed{,}$ $\boxed{\text{alpha}}$ $\boxed{\text{N}}$ $\boxed{,}$ 1 $\boxed{,}$ 5 $\boxed{)}$. Now press $\boxed{\text{ENTER}}$ to see a list of the first five terms of the sequence. The calculator is set in Auto mode, so the terms are expressed as fractions. In order to see the fifth term in the list we must first press $\boxed{\triangle}$ to move to the history area of the screen. Then we press $\boxed{\triangleright}$ repeatedly until the entire term can be seen.

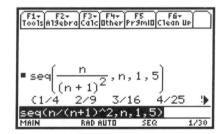   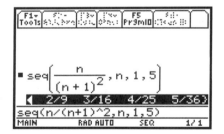

FINDING PARTIAL SUMS

We can use a graphing calculator to find partial sums of a sequence for which the general term is given by a formula.

Section 10.1, Example 5 Use a graphing calculator to find S_1, S_2, S_3, and S_4 for the sequence in which the general term is given by $a_n = (-1)^n/(n+1)$.

We will use the cumSum feature from the Math List menu. This option lists the cumulative, or partial, sums for a sequence defined using the Sequence feature discussed above. First use $\boxed{\triangledown}$ to highlight the current entry on the entry line of the home screen. Then copy cumSum to the entry line of the home screen by pressing $\boxed{\text{2nd}}$ $\boxed{\text{Math}}$ 3 7. Next copy the Sequence feature by pressing $\boxed{\text{2nd}}$ $\boxed{\text{Math}}$ 3 1. Now enter the general term of the sequence, the variable, and the first and last partial sums we wish to calculate, all separated by commas. Press $($ $(-)$ 1 $)$ $\wedge$ alpha N $\div$ $($ alpha N $+$ 1 $)$ $,$ alpha N $,$ 1 $,$ 4 $)$ $)$ ENTER . Note that we must use $\triangle$ to move to the history area of the screen and then press $\triangleright$ repeatedly until the entire fourth sum can be seen.

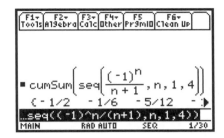 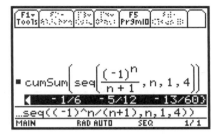

GRAPHS OF SEQUENCES

Section 10.1, Example 8 Graph the sequence for which the general term is given by $a_n = (-1)^n/n$.

The calculator must be set in Sequence mode to graph a sequence.

Press $\diamond$ $Y =$ to go to the sequence-editor screen, and enter $u1 = (-1)^n/n$ by positioning the cursor beside "$u1 =$" and pressing $($ $(-)$ 1 $)$ $\wedge$ alpha N $\div$ alpha N .

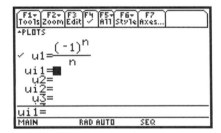

The domain of a sequence is a set of integers, so the graph of a sequence is a set of points that are not connected. Thus, we use Dot style to graph a sequence. Press $2nd$ $F6$ 2 to select "Dot" from the Style menu on the sequence-editor screen.

Next we enter the window dimensions. We will graph the sequence from $n = 1$ through $n = 15$, so we let nmin = 1, nmax = 15, xmin = 1, and xmax = 20. A table of values of the sequence shows that the terms appear to be between -1 and 1, so we let ymin = -1 and ymax = 1 with yscl = 0.1. We also set both plotStrt and plotStep to 1. These settings cause the graph to begin with the first term in the sequence and to plot each term of the sequence.

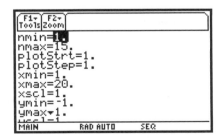 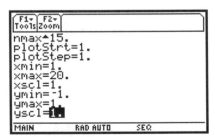

Press $\diamond$ | GRAPH | to see the graph of the sequence.

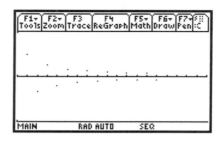

EVALUATING FACTORIALS

Factorials can be evaluated on a graphing calculator.

Section 10.4, Example 3 Simplify: $\dfrac{8!}{5!3!}$.

We use the factorial feature, denoted !, from the Math Probability menu. On the entry line of the home screen press 8 | 2nd |

| MATH | 7 1 | ÷ | | (| 5 | 2nd | | MATH | 7 1 3 | 2nd | | MATH | 7 1 |) | | ENTER |. Note that we must use parentheses in the denominator

so that 8! is divided by both 5! and 3!.

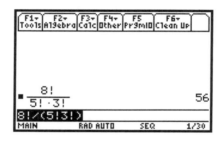

SIMPLIFYING $\left(\begin{array}{c} n \\ r \end{array} \right)$ NOTATION

Section 10.4, Example 4(a) Simplify: $\left(\begin{array}{c} 7 \\ 2 \end{array} \right)$.

The calculator uses the notation $_nC_r$ instead of $\left(\begin{array}{c} n \\ r \end{array} \right)$. To calculate $\left(\begin{array}{c} 7 \\ 2 \end{array} \right)$ on a TI-89 we use the $_nC_r$ feature from the

Probability submenu of the Math menu. On the TI-89, $_7C_2$ is entered as $_nC_r(7,2)$.

Press | 2nd | | MATH | 7 3 7 | , | 2 |) | | ENTER |. The first four keystrokes display the Math Probability menu and select item 3,

$_nC_r$, from that menu. The remaining keystrokes enter the values for n and r separated by a comma, close the expression with a

right parenthesis, and finally cause $_7C_2$ to be evaluated. The result is 21.

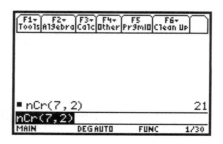

TI-83 and TI-83 Plus Index

Index
TI-86 Graphics Calculator

Index
TI-89 Graphics Calculator